African nurses and everyday work in twentieth-century Zimbabwe

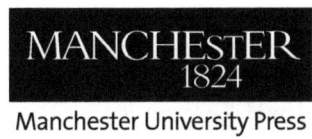

Manchester University Press

Nursing History and Humanities

Series editors: Christine E. Hallett and Jane E. Schultz

This series provides an outlet for the publication of rigorous academic texts in the two closely related disciplines of Nursing History and Nursing Humanities, drawing upon both the intellectual rigour of the humanities and the practice-based, real-world emphasis of clinical and professional nursing.

At the intersection of Medical History, Women's History and Social History, Nursing History remains a thriving and dynamic area of study with its own claims to disciplinary distinction. The broader discipline of Medical Humanities is of rapidly growing significance within academia globally, and this series aims to encourage strong scholarship in the burgeoning area of Nursing Humanities more generally.

Such developments are timely, as the nursing profession expands and generates a stronger disciplinary axis. The MUP Nursing History and Humanities series provides a forum within which practitioners and humanists may offer new findings and insights. The international scope of the series is broad, embracing all historical periods and including both detailed empirical studies and wider perspectives on the cultures of nursing.

Previous titles in this series:

Mental health nursing: The working lives of paid carers in the nineteenth and twentieth centuries
Edited by Anne Borsay and Pamela Dale

Negotiating nursing: British Army sisters and soldiers in the Second World War
Jane Books

One hundred years of wartime nursing practices, 1854–1953
Edited by Jane Brooks and Christine E. Hallett

'Curing queers': Mental nurses and their patients, 1935–74
Tommy Dickinson

Histories of nursing practice
Edited by Gerard M. Fealy, Christine E. Hallett and Susanne Malchau Dietz

Nurse writers of the Great War
Christine Hallett

Beyond Nightingale: Nursing on the Crimean War battlefields
Carol Helmstadter

Who cared for the carers? A history of the occupational health of nurses, 1880–1948
Debbie Palmer

Colonial caring: A history of colonial and post-colonial nursing
Edited by Helen Sweet and Sue Hawkins

Ellen N. La Motte: Nurse, writer, activist
Lea M. Williams

AFRICAN NURSES AND EVERYDAY WORK IN TWENTIETH-CENTURY ZIMBABWE

CLEMENT MASAKURE

Manchester University Press

Copyright © Clement Masakure 2020

The right of Clement Masakure to be identified as the author of this work has been asserted by them in accordance with the Copyright, Designs and Patents Act 1988.

Published by Manchester University Press
Altrincham Street, Manchester M1 7JA
www.manchesteruniversitypress.co.uk

British Library Cataloguing-in-Publication Data
A catalogue record for this book is available from the British Library

ISBN   978 1 5261 3547 6 hardback

First published 2020

The publisher has no responsibility for the persistence or accuracy of URLs for any external or third-party internet websites referred to in this book, and does not guarantee that any content on such websites is, or will remain, accurate or appropriate.

Typeset by Newgen Publishing UK

For my family

Contents

List of figures	viii
List of tables	ix
Acknowledgements	x
Map	xii

1	Introduction: African nurses in Zimbabwe's hospitals	1
2	The experiences of the pioneer generation of nurses, *c.* 1900–49	24
3	'Our kitchen days are over … We can no longer continue the tradition of our predecessors': Taking up nursing as a career option, *c.* 1950 to the 1960s	63
4	The Africanisation of Rhodesia's clinical spaces and an anatomy of everyday work in hospitals, 1960–70	94
5	Nursing a nation at war: Nurses' experiences during the 1970s	135
6	The trajectories of nursing in independent Zimbabwe, 1980–96	173
7	Conclusion: Nurses and nursing in twentieth-century Zimbabwe	214

Appendix 1: Colonial and post-colonial names	225
Appendix 2: Explanations and translations	226
Bibliography	227
Index	242

Figures

Every reasonable attempt has been made to obtain permission to reproduce copyright images. If any proper acknowledgement has not been made, copyright holders are invited to contact the author via Manchester University Press.

2.1	An early mission station clinic (courtesy National Archives of Zimbabwe)	32
2.2	Sr Madge Dry with some of the nurses she trained (194-) [Date incomplete] (courtesy National Archives of Zimbabwe)	38
2.3	A medical orderly treating a patient (courtesy National Archives of Zimbabwe)	45
2.4	An outdoor African clinic (courtesy National Archives of Zimbabwe)	47
4.1	Harare Hospital trainees (195-) [Date incomplete] (courtesy National Archives of Zimbabwe)	100
7.1	Treatment of leprosy (courtesy National Archives of Zimbabwe)	215

Tables

2.1	The number of nurses in training at mission stations (1943)	39
2.2	A summary of government clinics and patients treated between 1936 and 1946	42
3.1	Salaries per month: African student orderlies (1958)	82
3.2	Salaries: Trainee nurses (1958)	83
6.1	Total number of HIV/AIDS cases by year (national)	191

Acknowledgements

This book was made possible by the women and men who gave up their valuable time to share their stories with me. Their willingness to talk about their life experiences despite the tense political and harsh economic environment prevailing in Zimbabwe left me humbled. I would also like to thank the staff at the National Archives who, since the beginning of this project, made it possible for me to access invaluable archival documents and directed me to other material that I would have missed in the catalogues. Their assistance is much appreciated.

Over the course of writing the book, I have benefited a great deal from mentors and colleagues. At the University of Minnesota – Twin Cities, Allen Isaacman and Helena Pohlandt-McCormick were instrumental in shaping early ideas around this project. They provided a model of patience and commitment to one's work that will continue to inspire my own intellectual and professional development. I will forever be grateful. To my colleagues, Terrence Mashingaidze, Munya Munochiveyi, Ireen Mudeka, Jones Sichali, Oswald Masebo and Eleusio Phillipe, I am glad that our paths met and thank you for the sharp intellectual engagements.

At the University of the Free State, I would like to thank Ian Phimister for his untiring support and encouragement to complete this work. I am grateful for his support and guidance. Credit goes to Rosa Williams, Andy Cohen, Rory Pilosof, Daniel Spence, Kate Law, Jackie du Toit, Neil Roos and the rest of the ISG team, who provided sharp comments and critiques that went into shaping this work. A special thank you to Ilse le Roux and Tarisai Gwena for your kindness and hard work in making my further research easier during my time

Acknowledgements

with the ISG. Additionally, J. P Mtisi, P. S Nyambara. E. Kramer and A. Mlambo – my history lecturers at the University of Zimbabwe – your role in shaping my intellectual journey is duly appreciated.

I would like to further thank Manchester University Press for allowing me to contribute to their Nursing History Series, the two anonymous reviewers who took time to read the proposal and the drafts as well as the editors for their great patience in seeing this project through.

To my parents, who have been extremely supportive in all my endeavours and my siblings and their families, I thank you for your understanding and encouragement throughout this project. To my generous and loving wife Tarisai and to my daughter Anashe Chido and my son Avongwe Washe, my deepest gratitude for your multifaceted support. The three of you have generously filled a void in my life, you are so dearly loved.

Lastly, I take full responsibility for any shortcomings of this book.

This research was funded by The MacArthur Program – MacArthur and Compton Fellowships, University of Minnesota; University of Minnesota History Department; University of the Free State Post-doctoral Research Fellowship and the University of the Free State Prestige Scholars' Programme.

Map

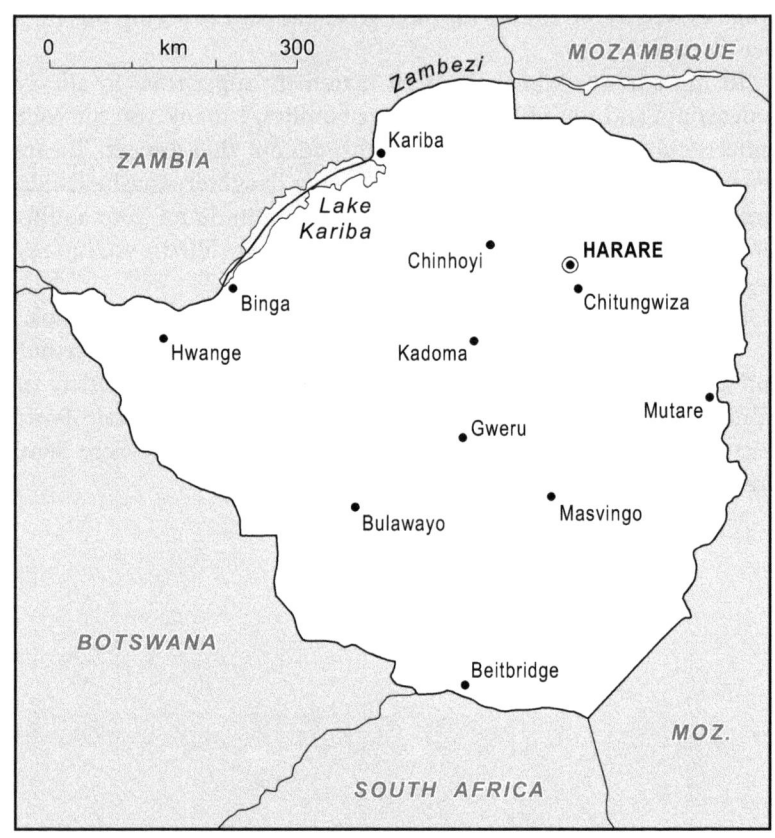

Map of Zimbabwe

1
Introduction: African nurses in Zimbabwe's hospitals

In 2008, at the height of the cholera epidemic in Zimbabwe, retired nurse Laiza Shumba visited a colleague who was working at Harare Hospital. What she saw there, as she put it, was a dire situation. The nurses were under-resourced and underpaid, and she knew they would not be able to fight the disease effectively without enough support from the authorities. In her interview with me a few weeks later, she observed that the modern nurse's plight raises challenges from the past to an entirely new and unforeseen level:

> I am not saying it was all rosy in the past. It was not! We had our own challenges during the colonial period and even in the early post-colonial era. However, I did not experience what the present day nurses are going through. To be honest, I feel sorry for them. If the situation continues like this, the profession will lose its prestige.[1]

At the intersection of nursing history and the history of hospitals in colonial and post-colonial societies, this book tells the story of Laiza Shumba and her generation of nurses who entered the profession in the post-1950 period. It also places the history of the earlier generations of hospital workers centre stage; those men and women who commenced hospital work in the first decade of the twentieth century. It is thus a story of the generations of African[2] nurses who practised their craft in hospitals for just over a century in the former British colony of Southern Rhodesia, now Zimbabwe.[3] In telling the story of these nurses, the book highlights nurses' experiences within and outside hospital spaces.

In the course of interviewing Zimbabwean nurses about their experiences, I noticed some recurring themes: nurses' struggles within hospitals, how African nurses constituted the backbone of the hospital system, their fight against disease (encapsulated in the phrase *tairwisa zvirerwe* – 'we were fighting illness/diseases'),[4] and the prestige associated with the profession. Nurses in Zimbabwe, to borrow from Rima Apple, 'played vital roles in the delivery of healthcare and shaping of colonial and post-colonial relations'.[5] Through nursing, African nurses shaped such colonial and post-colonial relations within and outside of hospitals. Hence, a history of nurses must not focus on work in hospitals alone, but also appreciate the influences and perceptions of nurses within African communities. Beyond clinical spaces, Africans held the profession in high esteem. However, the poor working conditions and inadequate remuneration, as Laiza Shumba's observations suggest, would over time come to erode the prestige associated with the profession.

My reconstruction of this story is organised around the following broad and interrelated questions. First, what were the experiences of African nurses working in Zimbabwe's hospitals in the twentieth century and how did their experiences change over time? Second, considering the hierarchical structure of colonial and post-colonial societies that was replicated in hospitals, as subordinates within the hierarchy, in what ways did African nurses transform these spaces to make them their own? Third, how did nurses themselves and society at large conceptualise the work of nursing? At one level, the questions framing this study enable us to examine the centrality of African nurses in the provision of care during the period under study. On another level, the questions allow us to peer into hospitals, enabling us to interrogate and flesh out nurses' everyday work experiences. In addition, the questions open up ways of understanding and disentangling the complex relations between nurses themselves as well as between nurses and their superiors. At the same time, the questions also enable us to move beyond hospitals, exploring what the profession offered to those who practised it and societal expectations of nurses. It is important to appreciate that nurses' struggles – within and outside clinical spaces – were part of the broader national struggles during the period under study.

Through an analytical lens that focuses on nurses' work and what comes with that work, the book teases out the experiences of practising nursing in hospitals. Henriette Moore reminds us that work is more than the exertion of physical activity by a person over material objects or, in the case of nurses, on patients. According to Moore 'the definition of work must also include the conditions under which that work is performed, and its perceived social values or worth within a given cultural context'.[6] African nurses were defined by their work. Within clinical spaces, their daily work and the nature of the work structured the relations between nurses and their superiors and amongst nurses. Outside hospital spaces, the nature of their profession (work) and the associated authority that came with it, affected their social standing within their community.

The hierarchical nature of the hospital institution conditioned nurses' work experiences. During the colonial period, race and gender informed experiences and relations. As a product of colonial bureaucracy, the structure and organisation of hospitals reflected colonial power relations, with white male administrators and medical doctors at the top of the pyramid, followed by white nurses, both senior and junior nurses. Coloured/Asian nurses followed in time. African nurses, nursing assistants and nursing orderlies anchored the bottom of the pyramid. The Africanisation of hospital administration that started in the later stages of colonial rule and ended in the immediate independent period, did little to change the structure of hospitals. Thus, colonial power relations extended beyond the post-colonial period. For the early years of independence, colonial power relations continued to inform relations between nurses and their superiors. Yet, within such an environment, African nurses carved out a niche for themselves and made workspaces (hospitals) their own. Indeed, not only were African nurses the backbone of nursing practice in colonial hospitals but, as demonstrated throughout the book, nursing practice within colonial hospitals gave African nurses an opportunity to reshape perceptions of nursing and the care economy during the period under study.

The book also underscores that, irrespective of their subordinate position within hospitals, nurses retained a degree of autonomy over the work process. This partial autonomy stemmed from the limits of nurses' superiors' supervision abilities and the very nature of the job. Hence, as much as nurses were under the supervision of doctors and/or matrons, having the knowledge and authority over important tasks, such as documenting patient conditions, diagnosing diseases and administering vaccines, allowed them a measure of autonomy in the practice of their work. The pioneer nurses were authorities in rural government clinics due to the relative absence of medical doctors in the countryside. The same can be said about the later generation of nurses who worked in urban hospitals in the second half of the twentieth century. Southern Rhodesia never managed to train enough white hospital workers during the period under study. This left African nurses in charge of hospitals and lent them a degree of autonomy when it came to nursing practice. A similar situation played itself out during the war of liberation in the 1970s, commonly known as the Second Chimurenga. The relative absence of senior medical personnel in the Rhodesian countryside in the 1970s at the height of the war gave nurses an opportunity to expand the scope of their practice, assert their autonomy and take responsibility of the rural clinic. This was not peculiar to Zimbabwe. The history of nursing in some parts of Africa demonstrates how nurses' work at times included responsibilities such as diagnosis and treatment; modalities that were not typical of nurses' everyday practice in Europe or the United States.[7] Being the last bastion of clinical medicine in rural areas, African nurses made more decisions than before as they experienced new levels of autonomy. The ability to control the work process, whether in rural or urban hospitals, provided nurses with a degree of control over their work and hospital spaces.

Sweet and Hawkins argued that nursing history opens up ways of interrogating cultural differences.[8] As in other parts of the colonial world, indigenous nurses were critical bridges between the colonisers and the colonised in dispensing biomedicine. As 'middles',[9] to borrow from Nancy Rose Hunt, African nurses in Zimbabwe were significant cultural brokers, who, as Anne Digby and Helen Sweet showed in the case of missionary nurses in South Africa, were 'between the "modern" western medical model of their training and the African traditional medicine of their patients'.[10] In addition, Hunt noted that the acceptance of colonial medicine 'was mediated by the new colonial categories of middles and the "entangled objects" of their work'.[11] Following Hunt, Digby, Sweet and others, this book also posits that, as cultural interlocutors, African nurses in Zimbabwe translated African conceptions of affliction to white medical personnel and simultaneously translated biomedicine to African patients. In fact, the establishment and running of early Christian Mission hospitals depended on the assistance of the in-house trained pioneer generation of nurses. This generation bridged the divide between white hospital workers and African patients in the early years of colonial rule. During the first decade of the twentieth century, early converts such as Tizora M. Neves received great praise in missionary records for their role in bridging the cultural divide between missionaries and African patients and in establishing missionary medical work amongst African communities. In the 1920s, Dr Gurney, a missionary doctor, was frustrated by what he perceived as Africans' failure to use western remedies. He was also agitated by 'many natives who cannot describe conditions with sufficient accuracy to enable a correct diagnosis'.[12] The success of Gurney's work rested on the assistance he received from Job Tsiga. Furthermore, from the 1930s onwards, the government-trained Advanced Male Native Nursing Orderlies, as well as the formal Christian Mission-trained female nurses, continued the tradition. Both categories of nurses were products of the government's introduction of rural clinics together with the missionaries' quest for more formal training of nurses within their hospitals. Over a significant part of the period, African nurses continued to be cultural interlocutors. In the late 1970s and early 1980s, the problem of African patients' incapacity to describe afflictions according to western standards continued.[13] Flora Matondo recollected that many patients explained illness through the cultural framework. For example, claiming that illness is due to *chipotswa*: an affliction characterised by the sensation of an object moving rhythmically from one part of the body to another, e.g. from the left ear to the right groin. Other patients claimed that their affliction was a result of *kuroyiwa* (bewitchment). The patients who explained illness through a cultural framework nevertheless sought western medical help.[14] This was frustrating to health personnel. The problem was not Africans' so-called incapacity to explain affliction, rather, the predicament rested on cultural differences and the language employed in explaining illness and disease causation. Because many white doctors and nursing personnel lacked the grammar to articulate and understand the afflicted, they ended up relying chiefly on African nurses to translate the nature of the illness. In this process, therefore, African nurses drew upon cultural norms of disease causation, health and healing. Tapping into and co-opting cultural understandings of therapy in hospitals enabled them to transform hospitals into spaces that showed their expertise and transformed the hospital spaces into their own. In addition, by drawing from African cultural healing repertoires, African nurses came to terms with colonial medicine and reformulated local ideas of healing and nursing.

The manner in which the hospital functioned changed Africans' understanding of health and healing just as young women nursing older, male patients did. Many came to terms with the idea of having access to strangers' bodies. Tsitsi Chinamasa recollected that during her years as a student nurse, she felt uncomfortable requesting older male patients to undress for examinations. Bathing older men made her uncomfortable.[15] Patients themselves also felt uneasy being instructed to undress or to have their bodies checked by younger nurses. In the 1960s at Harari Central Hospital, authorities discovered that older men were slow in recovering due to their reluctance to disclose the nature of their ailments to young nurses. It is a belief within the Shona/Ndebele culture that a patient is not supposed to reveal his/her illness to strangers.[16] The patients found it difficult to divulge their ailments to women similar in age to their daughters or daughters in law. To this end, women's work provides an opportunity to examine the health transformations that took place among Africans with the introduction of hospitals.

Based on the experiences of hospital nurses, providing care – in what nurses conceptualised as – *kuriswa zvirwere* (fighting diseases/illness) and *kupepa varwere* (nursing the infirm), my study goes far beyond the anecdotal. The history of nursing, I contend, must move beyond hospital walls to examine African nurses within colonial and post-colonial communities. An examination of nurses' experiences beyond the clinical space makes visible the social transformations that took place in colonial Zimbabwe during the time under study. Women constitute the majority of nurses in Zimbabwe. Therefore, the study of nurses in Zimbabwe is incomplete if it fails to examine African women's hopes and aspirations in taking up nursing. One of the central arguments I make is that because the government preferred to train female nurses, opening up nursing to African women, we must take note that these women were important historical actors who chose nursing for various reasons. Amongst other things, nursing offered new possibilities for African women who were living in a racist and patriarchal society. African women saw nursing as an avenue to secure a better life for themselves and their families. Employment opportunities through nursing contributed to the sudden and unprecedented rise in these women's social positions. Becoming members of the new African middle class marked a change in the self-perceptions of those who worked as nurses. In the past, their fathers and subsequently their husbands primarily determined women's positions within society. As nurses, women's social standing was also identified by their achievement and by the degree of independence they acquired apart from male control.[17]

In addition, with the extension of the State Registered Nursing (SRN) programme to African women in the post-1945 period, nursing took on a different meaning for most of the women who joined the profession. It was more than a job. Africans, in this case, women, just as the earlier generation of hospital workers, took the opportunity to highlight their abilities in a racist and oppressive society. Because education was restricted for Africans in general and African women in particular, only a small number of women could qualify to enter the nursing programme. For those women, nursing was more than just everyday work; it represented what African women could achieve if given an opportunity. African nurses, as veteran nationalist Edison Sithole wrote, epitomised the progress of African people living under tough circumstances.[18] For African women, nursing contributed to African society just as white nurses, who left the United Kingdom, did so to help Britain's colonies.[19] In short, privileging women's motives for choosing nursing as a preferred, though limited, career option, prompts analysis of the social and economic changes that took place amongst African women in colonial Zimbabwe.

Centring on nurses' work and the nature of the work process brings into focus hospitals and their culture. Nursing historian Barbara Melosh pointed out that such culture has specific language, tradition and social rules that workers (nurses) create on the job. Hence, terms like work culture, shop floor culture and occupational culture suggest coherence and structure in activities.[20] This occupational culture is central in guiding and interpreting the tasks and social relations of work. Furthermore, workplace culture 'embodies workers' definition of a good day's work, their measure of satisfying competent performance'.[21] Melosh further argued that nursing's occupational culture, a product of nurses' distinctive training, 'provided the lore, the anecdote, and the prescription for managing the nurse's intricate gender and race-based relationships with patients, doctors, supervisors, and administrators'.[22] In this study, workplace relationships are important in analysing the experiences of nurses within clinical spaces. Nursing scholars have shown how nursing illuminates the way in which gender informs work and how this work reproduces and transforms relationships of power and inequality.[23] Undoubtedly, labour division within hospitals replicated a larger sexual division of labour. Caring for patients imitated the relationship of a mother and children; deference to doctors was structured similarly to women's deference to fathers and husbands. Even the relationship between junior nurses and their superiors was framed within paternalistic relationships in a hospital system that privileged senior women.

These gendered and feminised ideas were transplanted to the colonies with the introduction of western hospitals and biomedicine. In settler societies such as Rhodesia and South Africa, the hospital system replicated larger racial and class divisions of labour. For South Africa, Belinda Bozzoli and Shula Marks pointed out that the cleavages along gender lines mirrored race and class divisions. Hence, relationships of domination and subordination were not just a result of inequalities between different races and classes in South Africa; there were also inequalities among men and women, and white, coloured and black women.[24] According to Marks, power relations 'were made more complex by racial, ethnic and class divisions within the profession while the form that professionalism took reinforced racial and class cleavages'.[25] Rhodesian clinical spaces followed a similar trajectory with a fractured sisterhood informed by race and class.

Historiographical context

Considering that there is very little historical work on nursing in Zimbabwe,[26] *African nurses and everyday work in twentieth-century Zimbabwe* takes up the challenge set by Helen Sweet and Sue Hawkins in *Colonial caring: A history of colonial and post-colonial nursing*.[27] Sweet and Hawkins noted that while nursing history has shifted in its examining of professionalisation within national borders by employing a more strongly international emphasis, there is still a gap within nursing history around the role that nurses and nursing played in a country's past. More specifically, the book's starting point constitutes the work of nursing historians who have not only examined the various ways in which nursing and hospitals became sites of race, class, and gender and ethnic struggles, but also focused on nurses who occupied the lower rungs of the profession, in the process giving voice to those silenced in nursing historiography.[28] In Rhodesia, African nurses were in a subordinate position within hospitals. Even when some of them were elevated to senior positions in the second half of the twentieth century, colonial relations dictated nurses' daily experiences. Despite their subordinate position, indigenous nurses played a significant role in administrating biomedicine. As Megan Vaughan persuasively argued, biomedicine was practised not only on Africans but also by Africans.[29] At the same time, African nurses translated and negotiated biomedicine to African patients. In the process, such personnel incorporated local practices and appropriated local concepts to fit biomedical practices.[30] While this book examines African nurses' everyday work within hospitals, it also emphasises nurses' experiences beyond the confines of the hospital. In doing so, the book expands upon Horwitz's examination of the diverse motives for choosing nursing as a career,[31] and relates childhood experiences with nursing, a neglected connection within nursing history.

The Zimbabwean case gives nursing history an opportunity to make comparison with South Africa. In fact, the history of nursing in Zimbabwe mirrors some of the key developments of nursing history in South Africa. While Rhodesia enticed health administrators from the United Kingdom, a significant proportion of white nurses and government officials who occupied influential positions in South Africa migrated to Rhodesia. In their various capacities, they brought ideologies that influenced the practice of nursing in the colony. As noted earlier, racial identities in colonial Zimbabwe, as in South Africa, affected the very nature of relations amongst nurses working in hospitals during the colonial period. An equally crucial analytical tool is gender. Like South Africa, the majority of nurses in Zimbabwe are women. Indeed, up to a particular point in South African and Zimbabwean nursing histories, men, who at times were not classified as nurses within the records, provided nursing services to their fellow Africans. In Zimbabwe, as demonstrated in the book, male nursing orderlies made up the spine of rural clinics in the pre-1950s era. In the 1970s, male guerrilla medics provided nursing services to civilians and combatants at the height of the liberation struggle. Yet, there was no formal training of male nurses until 1966.[32] Even with the training of the few males as nurses starting in 1966, the presence of a formally trained male nurse within hospitals was an exception to the rule. This comes out of the nature of colonialism experienced in colonial settler societies such as Zimbabwe and South Africa. As in South Africa, the presence of women in clinical spaces in Zimbabwe was a result of ideologies of the day that drove home an idea of nursing as an extension of the domestic economy. Thus, in Rhodesia, as in South Africa, the impetus for training African female nurses originated from racist attitudes towards patient care.[33] This saw the marginalisation of male nurses within Zimbabwean hospitals, and the dearth of male nurses in Zimbabwe mirrored closely what happened in South Africa.[34]

Unlike nursing history in South Africa, the Zimbabwean case allows us to interrogate the experiences of the same nurses at the time of the decolonisation process. The decolonisation process violently pitted African nationalists and the Rhodesian government against each other. In the 1970s, hospitals became sites of struggles that were also being fought in the political arena. For example, the racial conflicts within hospitals during the 1970s reflected the tensions and anxieties that gripped the nation at war. Besides accentuating racial tensions in hospitals, the war directly affected the provision of health services and the war affected urban and rural healthcare workers in various ways. Although urban healthcare workers coped with patient upsurges and workload increases, rural workers, those in the theatre of the struggle, bore the brunt of the war. Rural nurses juggled different belligerent armies, which eventually led to significant changes in nursing practice. They also dealt with patients suffering from war-inflicted injuries, a situation for which they were not trained. The presence of guerrilla camps brought further transformation in nursing practice at the height of the decolonisation process. Having limited trained nurses to nurse the infirm within guerrilla and refugee camps, the liberation movements relied on

Introduction

rudimentarily trained medics. The medical centres within camps – the 'bush hospitals' – were poorly funded. In spite of limited resources, nurses and medics manning 'bush hospitals' played a vital role in the provision of care to freedom fighters and refugees. From those who worked in urban and rural hospitals to those who operated the 'bush hospitals', nurses projected their work as more than just a profession; they saw it as their contribution to the liberation struggles. They were nursing a nation at war. This is a challenge to the way in which the war narratives have been employed and deployed by the ruling ZANU-PF party. By highlighting the significant role nurses played during the liberation war, this book thus challenges the tendency by political elites to marginalise and trivialise contributions of non-war veterans to the independence of Zimbabwe.

In addition, the book also moves beyond the colonial period by mapping the continuities and changes in everyday nursing work in the post-colonial era. The end of colonial rule was significant to Zimbabwe. The new socialist-oriented government took various steps to deracialise, democratise and expand the health delivery system by opening up hospitals to all Zimbabweans irrespective of their race and through promoting more Africans into senior positions within hospital administration. However, it was not all rosy. Despite the government's success, efforts at improving working conditions met numerous hurdles. The situation took a turn in the early 1990s when the government implemented austerity measures as the HIV/AIDS epidemic began to take root. The economic constraints and the new disease environment placed new burdens on nurses. In response, nurses deployed various coping mechanisms to cushion themselves from the challenges they faced. Being on the frontline of fighting illness and diseases – *kurwisa zvirwere* – nurses found ways to continue practising their craft, even though they were working under difficult conditions.

Sources and methods

In *African nurses and everyday work in twentieth-century Zimbabwe*, I integrate archival material and oral sources in weaving the history of African nurses. Produced by various actors at different historical periods, these sources complement each other. I use archival material from the National Archives of Zimbabwe located in Harare. The archive is the key repository that holds material on the development and provision of health services during the colonial period. The documents include the Medical Director's annual Public Health Reports from 1911 to 1978 and the Minister of Health's yearly Public Health Reports covering the period 1990–96. Also included in these documents are annual reports from the Chief Native Commissioner, the key government officials dealing with African (Native) Affairs in Rhodesia. The Chief Native Commissioner's reports cover the period up to the late 1930s. I also accessed a few files dealing with Salisbury Hospital in the 1930s.[35] The National Archives of Zimbabwe also have a file from the Southern Rhodesia Nurses' Association, which was significant in allowing me an interior view of white nurses' frustrations and working conditions in Rhodesian hospitals from the late 1930s to the mid-1940s.[36] I also consulted the African University Archives, a repository of missionary records of the United Methodist Church in Mutare. Together, these archival materials helped me in constructing the early colonial disease environment and gave me a glimpse into government and Christian Mission medical facilities up to the 1940s. This enabled me to reconstruct the world of the pioneer generation of African nurses.

The National Archives of Zimbabwe also house the evidence supplied to and the report of the National Health Services Commission of 1945. The Commission was set up to investigate *inter alia* the provision of an organised National Health Service in conformity with the modern conception of 'Health' which would ensure adequate medical, dental, nursing and hospital services for all the people of Southern Rhodesia.[37] Spanning all parts of the country, the Commission sought information through direct interviews and correspondence with medical doctors, hospital administrators, native commissioners, industrialists and council officials. By conducting a careful reading of the evidence supplied to the Commission, one gets an idea of the provision of nursing services in Rhodesia in the 1940s. One can also glean the prejudices against training African male nurses. Some of the recommendations from the Commission were responsible for setting in motion the changes that were to occur within nursing services in Rhodesia in the 1950s.

Introduction

Important as archival sources are in reconstructing the narratives of African nurses, these sources have their limitations. As products of colonial officials, colonial archives are cultural artefacts that 'erase certain kinds of knowledge, select some and valorise others', as Fredrick Cooper and Anne Stoler have argued.[38] Thus, in reading colonial archives, one must be cognisant of the nature of their production, how the intersection of, *inter alia*, race, class, gender and position within colonial hierarchy influenced what was privileged and what was hidden or silenced. For example, in the process of gathering evidence, the Commission gave less attention to African voices. In an extensive body of evidence that covered close to 400 pages of interviews together with numerous appendices of correspondence, direct evidence from Africans covered less than five pages.

Furthermore, conspicuous by their absence from those five pages were African women's voices. In colonial Zimbabwe, no matter their age, African women were treated as minors. Thus, African women's concerns and grievances were channelled through men. In this case, African women's anxieties about health issues and the possibilities of becoming fully trained nurses were conveyed through middle-class males who dominated organisations like the Bulawayo Bantu Community Association.[39] Thus, it is a big task to tease out from archival documents the experiences of Africans within colonial hospitals and the perspectives of African nurses' daily work. I read these documents from the colonial period carefully and critically, 'against the grain',[40] to retrieve the voices and agency of African nurses.

To address these challenges, I turned to African newspapers and magazines. Examples include *The African Parade*, *The African Weekly*, *The African Daily News* and *The Bantu Mirror*. Written by Africans, these newspapers span more than forty years. Newspapers opened a window through which I drew Africans' perceptions of health policy, the state of clinics in urban as well as rural areas, and their perceptions of African nurses. While African newspapers and magazines mainly focused on politics, they also included articles that examined the significance of nursing to African women, and the conduct that was expected of nurses. I read these newspapers with a critical eye as to how gender and class mediated perceptions of nursing. For their insights, newspapers muzzle the voices of

African nurses and instead reveal the biases of their writers and intended audiences. Written in English by male 'middle-class' writers and intended for the literate few, they projected their 'middle-class', patriarchal ethos in their discussions on nursing. Nevertheless, these sources complement the archival evidentiary base in constructing the story of African nurses from the colonial period into the post-colonial era.

Oral accounts form the principal evidence for this study. Initial interviews for this project were conducted between 2008 and 2009. Economically, this was a time of hyperinflation, and politically, the situation was tense.[41] At the same time, the public health system was in a shambles, and in August of 2008, Zimbabwe experienced one of the worst cholera outbreaks in the history of the nation.[42] Close to thirty female and male nurses in Harare and Mutare were interviewed. While two interviews were conducted by a colleague, I personally conducted the rest of the interviews. The interviewees' ages ranged from those in their mid to late fifties to those in their late seventies. Option for anonymity was made available but all the informants chose that their names be used for the study. In my hometown of Mutare it was not difficult to make connections, as some of the senior nurses are my neighbours and relations. For those who felt uncomfortable/unwilling to talk to me, they directed me to other nurses, and this gesture was critical in building trust between myself and the informant, considering the tense political situation at the time of the research. In Harare, I went to the premier institutions of Parirenyatwa and Harare hospitals. However, because of the volatile political situation and the cholera pandemic that made Zimbabwean hospitals a subject of international media, some of my informants were unwilling to be interviewed at work. Considering that the government was downplaying cholera cases and the dire conditions of hospitals in the country and labelling anyone who spoke publicly against health policies an enemy of the state, I assured them that I was not a journalist working for an international organisation and that their responses would be used only for academic purposes.

The interviews were mainly conducted in the vernacular Shona, though there were many cases of language switching between Shona and English. Language switching is common in Zimbabwe. Interviewees agreed to use their names, most of the interviews were recorded, and I translated them into English. When conducting interviews, I was aware of my positionality as a male researcher especially when interviewing female nurses and coming from an American university.

Some of the nurses I approached for interviews were surprised that I was conducting such research as they reminded me that there were many other political events that I could write on. Others indicated that they never thought that one could write a history of nurses or even think about the history of hospitals and diseases. For them, history was what they were taught at school, about political events and big names or, as Estella Dhlamini indicated, 'history of the war veterans and the war we see every day on Zimbabwe National TV'.[43] In most cases, I took the time to assure them that their life stories are also part of Zimbabwean history.

By stressing the importance of oral histories in the reconstruction of Zimbabwean nurses' history, I am following in the footsteps of social historians. What I noticed is that older nurses were eager to emphasise their childhood experiences and these were instrumental in influencing them to enter the nursing profession. They reminded me of the problems and difficulties they faced as young women during the colonial era and how the situation has changed in the post-colonial era. Nurses also underscored their struggles with their superiors and how they worked hard in nursing the sick. For instance, when Phaina Nyanhanda was interviewed about her daily work, she replied that, 'We worked very hard but I think it was very good for us for we took care of patients better than nurses of today. I think we were patient oriented but today's nurses are book oriented.'[44] Others complained about today's nurses as uncaring, good at gossiping and interested in money:

> These young nurses do not focus on their work. They are more interested in gossiping and talking about today's fashions. You hear them talking about the latest hairstyles working in the wards. We would do these things during our spare time and not when you have patients to take care of.[45]

What is fascinating to note is that information from newspapers in the 1960s mentions similar problems amongst nurses. A 1961 letter to *The African Weekly* suggested that nurses 'misbehave with their boyfriends, are lazy [they] do not know how to keep their homes clean, nurses worry about money and getting married to rich people and so on'.[46] In the early 1980s, there were numerous reports of uncaring, petulant and money-loving nurses.[47] On the other hand, younger nurses underscored their dedication to the profession and the need to serve their community by taking care of the infirm:

> These days [at the time of the interviews], because of the problems and frustrations being experienced in the profession, many of our seniors quickly point fingers at junior nurses. Young women have so many options open to them but the fact that they chose nursing is an indicator [of] their commitment to the profession.[48]

To account for these contrasting narratives, I considered generational differences and what it meant to be a nurse in post-colonial Zimbabwe. There was a tendency for older nurses to romanticise the past, even when they experienced racial discrimination. For instance, most of the older nurses argued that even though their salaries were lower in comparison to their coloured/Asian and white counterparts, '*yakanga iri mari kwayo. Taitozviotengera zvinhu zvedu* (wages were reasonable. We managed to buy valuable commodities)'.[49] In trying to come to terms with this romanticisation of the past, I was reminded of Michel-Rolph Trouillot's words: 'the past does not exist independent of the present ... the past is only the past because there is a present'.[50] In other words, the past is not hermetically sealed from the present. Rather the present shapes historical understandings of the past. As most of my informants articulated their clinical experiences in detail, it was clear that most eagerly shared their stories with me because they were disappointed with the state of hospitals at the time of interviews. The economic and political situation in 2008 to 2009 further led to frustrations.

On the economic side, Zimbabwe was experiencing the highest inflation in the world, with civil servants failing to access even their inflated salaries in banks. On the political front, the environment was tense following the aftermath of the March 2008 elections and the runoff in June that saw massive intimidation of opposition supporters in both urban and rural areas. Furthermore, Zimbabwe's public health system was in a state of paralysis. While the provision of health services had been matching the economic decline starting in the 1990s, it was clear by 2006 that the health sector was in a shambles. Burdened

Introduction

with mounting HIV/AIDS cases, tuberculosis and malnutrition, the decline in health services was accelerated by the government's failure to reinvest in public health infrastructure. With the shortage of foreign currency, it became tough for the government to procure drugs. Slowly, hospitals turned into 'mortuaries,' as Estella Dhlamini claimed.[51] In fact, between September and November 2008, some hospital wards in the main public hospitals gradually closed due to shortages of personnel, drug shortages and general neglect. The most abrupt halt in healthcare access occurred on 17 November 2008, when the premier teaching and referral hospital in Harare, Parirenyatwa, closed along with the medical school.[52] To make matters worse, between August 2008 and March 2009, nurses were trying to come to terms with the cholera outbreak. All these factors were important in reminding me that the various ways in which nurses interpreted and projected the past was a political act meant to make a critique of their situation at the time of the research. As Tamara Giles-Vernick warned us, in dealing with oral sources we have to be attentive to the fact that 'our informants filter such interpretations through their perceptions of contemporary personal, social, political and economic relations.'[53] In an environment that made many reluctant to speak against the government for fear of retribution from '*vana takwarwa hondo*' (liberation war veterans),[54] the romanticisation and glorification of the past were framed by the realities within clinical spaces at the time of the research.

Another challenge of retrieving and using these memories is the inherent silences that are typical of any set of oral sources. Oral historians have demonstrated that silences are part of the everyday practice of memory, and any set of historical memories are particular bundles of silences. I became aware of the silences in my informants' responses when almost all the interviews I conducted were silent on detailed information on sexually transmitted diseases and birthing practices within clinical spaces. These issues were only addressed in passing references. My own positionality as a male Zimbabwean contributed to these passing remarks. In a situation where most of my informants were elders, some of whom I personally knew, I was culturally assigned the position of a son and a *munyarikani*. Within the Shona culture, a *munyarikani* is a person with whom one has a very close relationship but cannot discuss matters related to sex and sexuality. To do this, one relies on a *vana tete* (aunt), *sekuru* (uncle) or *sawhira* (close friend). It was impolite for me to ask about sexually transmitted diseases or about the changes in the birthing process as I was reminded of my positionality as a son and male. For example, Nomsa Makoni was talking about her anxiety with male bodies, especially those suffering from *zvirwerwe zvepabonde* (sexually transmitted diseases). Upon my probing for further details, she quickly reminded me that, 'you know these diseases and I cannot tell you anything more than what I have said'.[55] Despite their problems, oral histories provided me with the interior view of the nurses' world during the colonial and post-colonial period. Information from interviews described the struggles they endured to enter the profession, their conceptual understanding of nursing, and their daily experiences in clinical spaces. They emphasised the tensions with their superiors and their problems with patients. While they experienced numerous problems, nurses stressed that they had no regrets taking up the profession. As Laiza Shumba highlighted, if given a chance, she would take up nursing again: 'I would still take up nursing because I love the job. You know, since I retired in 1999, I have always been on standby, coming back on several occasions to help with the staffing situation at the hospital. It is something that I have always wanted to do, and I am glad I had the chance to do this.'[56] Laiza Shumba spoke for many. Her life history is emblematic of the many nurses who since the 1950s have been on the front line of caring, shouldering the burden of nursing the nation. In short, despite the limitations and difficulties of interpretation, oral accounts constitute a substantial body of evidence on the experiences of nurses working in government hospitals during the time under study. As with other sources, oral accounts must be read carefully and critically.

What comes out of the sources described above, and out of deploying various methodologies, is a story of African nurses within Zimbabwean hospitals. The story brings out the experiences of African nurses – female and male – in the provision of services to African patients for a period covering close to a century. It starts in the 1900s, with the introduction of the colonial hospital system and ends in 1996, when nurses went on strike. This was the largest strike in the history of Zimbabwe and a key turning point in nursing history in Zimbabwe. Nevertheless, for us to appreciate the story of struggles,

Introduction

resilience and creativity in adapting to their subordinate position within hospitals that culminated in the largest strike in nursing history in Zimbabwe, one has to go back to the pioneer generation of nurses who, as noted in the next chapter, set in motion the African presence within clinical spaces as workers, and laid the foundation for future generations of nurses.

Notes

1 Interview: Mrs Laiza Shumba, Mabelreign Harare, 26 October 2008.
2 By African, I refer to black people of African descent as it was used in the archives to denote such people. I have to emphasise that white Zimbabweans are not categorised 'Africans' in this study because the various archival records, even those written by colonial officials and the day-to-day usage of the term 'African', clearly outlined blacks as Africans and not any other group of people. It is from this semantic context that the term is used. The terms 'white' and 'European' are used to refer to people of European origin. I use these two terms interchangeably. The term 'coloured' refers to people of mixed race while the term 'Asian' is used to refer to people of Asian origin.
3 In this book, I use colonial place names for the period under colonial rule. Post-colonial names are used for the post-colonial period and current names are in brackets: Southern Rhodesia/Rhodesia (Zimbabwe), Northern Rhodesia (Zambia), Salisbury (Harare), Gwelo (Gweru).
4 In the vernacular Shona language, *chirwere/urwere* is the word for disease or a condition of sickness and it is derived from the phrase *kurwa* – to fight. See H. Aschwanden (in collaboration with the African nursing sisters of Musiso Hospital, Zimbabwe), *Symbols of death: An analysis of the conscious of the Karanga* (Gweru: Mambo Press, 1987), p. 13.
5 R. Apple, 'Afterword', in H. Sweet and S. Hawkins (eds), *Colonial caring: A history of colonial and post-colonial nursing* (Manchester: Manchester University Press, 2015), p. 233.
6 H. Moore quoted in S. Rubert, *A most promising weed: A history of tobacco farming and labor in colonial Zimbabwe, 1890–1945* (Cleveland: Ohio University Press, 1998), p. xii.
7 See for example, B. Mann Wall, *Into Africa: A transnational history of Catholic medical missions and social change* (New Brunswick, NJ: Rutgers University Press, 2015), p. 45 and H. Sweet, 'Mission nursing in South African context: The spread of knowledge during the colonial and apartheid eras', in E. Fleischmann, S. Grypma, M. Marten, I. M. Okkenhaug (eds), *Transnational and historical perspectives on global health, welfare and humanitarianism* (Kristiansand: Portal Forlag Publishers, 2013), pp. 137–57.

8 Sweet and Hawkins (eds), *Colonial caring*, p. 1.
9 N. R. Hunt, *A colonial lexicon: Of birth ritual, medicalization, and mobility in the Congo* (Durham, NC: Duke University Press, 1999), p. 2.
10 A. Digby and H. Sweet, 'Nurses as culture brokers in twentieth-century South Africa', in W. Ernst (Ed.), *Plural medicine, tradition and modernity, 1800–2000* (London and New York: Routledge, 2002), pp. 113–29.
11 Hunt, *A colonial lexicon*, p. 2.
12 Africa University Archives: The Last Report of Dr Samuel Gurney to the Rhodesian Mission Conference, United Methodist Church, 19–26 June 1923.
13 O. M. Munyaradzi and C. Muronda, 'Some attitudes of patients discharged from Harare Hospital', *Central African Journal of Medicine*, 25: 5 (1979), pp. 104–7 and B. J. Kavumbura and R. T. Mossop, 'Attitudes to illness in Salisbury, 1980', *Central African Journal of Medicine*, 26: 5 (1980), pp. 111–14.
14 Interview: Mrs Flora Matondo, Sakubva Mutare, 12 August 2008.
15 Interview: Ms Tsitsi Chinamasa, Old Mutare Mission, 28 May 2009.
16 Interview: Kufa Mutoro, Mutare, 12 August 2008.
17 Interview: Mrs Phaina Nyanhanda, Harare, 15 August 2007. Interviewed by P. Mukwambo. For more on the struggles against patriarchal control see for example, E. Schmidt, *Peasants, traders, and wives: Shona women in the history of Zimbabwe* (Portsmouth, NH: Heinemann, 1992).
18 *The African Parade*, November 1958.
19 For colonial Zimbabwe see for example, C. Masakure, ' "One of the most serious problems confronting us at present": Nurses and government hospitals in Southern Rhodesia, 1930s to 1950', *Historia*, 60: 2 (2015), pp. 109–31.
20 B. Melosh, *The physician's hand: Work, culture and conflict in American nursing* (Philadelphia, PA: Temple University Press, 1982), p. 5.
21 Melosh, *The physician's hand*, p. 6.
22 Melosh, *The physician's hand*, p. 7.
23 See for example, E. Garmarnikow, 'Sexual division of labor: The case of nursing', in A. Kuhn and A. M. Wolpe (eds), *Feminism and materialism: Women and modes of production* (London: Boston and Henley, 1978), pp. 96–123; C. Davies, *Gender and the professional predicament of nursing* (Buckingham, UK: Open University Press, 1996) and S. Reverby, *Ordered to care: The dilemma of American nursing, 1850–1945* (New York: Cambridge University Press, 1987).
24 B. Bozzoli, 'Marxism, feminism and Southern African Studies', *Journal of Southern African Studies*, 9: 2 (1983), pp. 139–71.
25 S. Marks, *Divided sisterhood: Race, class and gender in the South African nursing profession* (London: St Martin's Press, 1994), pp. 3–4.
26 For a few historical works written on nurses and nursing in Zimbabwe see I. Mhike, 'A perennial shortage: State Registered Nurse training and recruitment in Southern Rhodesia's government hospitals, 1939–1963' (MA dissertation, University of Zimbabwe, 2007); C. Govha, 'A study of the implications

of racial and gender prejudices on African women in the nursing profession in colonial Zimbabwe, 1890-1960' (BA Honours dissertation, University of Zimbabwe, 2001); R. Charumbira, 'Administering medicine without a license: missionary women in Rhodesia's nursing history, 1890-1901', *The Historian*, 68: 2 (2006), pp. 241-66 and Masakure, 'One of the most serious problems confronting us at present'. Other works that are not historical but are also significant to consider are R. Gaidzanwa, *Voting with their feet: Migrant Zimbabwean nurses and doctors in the era of Structural Adjustment* (Uppsala: Nordiska Afrikainstitutet, 1999); A. Chikanda, 'Nurse migration from Zimbabwe: Analysis of recent trends and impacts', *Nursing Inquiry*, 12: 3 (2005), pp. 162-74 and J. McGregor, 'Professionals relocating: Zimbabwean nurses and teachers negotiating work and family in Britain', Geographical Paper, 178 (2006).

27 Sweet and Hawkins (eds), *Colonial caring*, p. 1.
28 Marks, *Divided sisterhood*; S. Marks, ' "We were men nursing men": Male nursing on the mines in twentieth-century South Africa', in W. Woodward, P. Hayes and G. Minkley (eds), *Deep histories: Gender and colonialism in Southern Africa* (Amsterdam: Rodipi, 2002) pp. 177-204; C. Burns, ' "A man is a clumsy thing who does not know how to handle a sick person": Aspects of the history of masculinity and race in the shaping of male nursing in South Africa, 1900-1950', *Journal of Southern African Studies*, 24: 4 (1998), pp. 695-717 and S. Horwitz, *Baragwanath Hospital Soweto: A history of medical care 1941-1990* (Johannesburg: Wits University Press, 2013), pp. 119-60. See also Melosh, *The physician's hand*; Reverby, *Ordered to care*; D. Clark Hine, *Black women in white: Racial conflict and cooperation in the nursing profession, 1890-1950* (Bloomington: Indiana University Press, 1989); S. L. Smith, *Sick and tired of being sick and tired: Black women's health activism in America, 1890-1950* (Philadelphia: University of Pennsylvania Press, 1995); V. N. Gamble, *Making a place for ourselves: The black hospital movement, 1920-1945* (Oxford: Oxford University Press, 1995) and C. C. Choy, *Empire of care: Nursing and migration in Filipino American History* (Durham, NC and London: Duke University Press, 2003).
29 M. Vaughan, *Curing their ills: Colonial power and African illness* (Stanford, CA: Stanford University Press, 1991), p. 64.
30 J. Turrittin, 'Colonial midwives and modernizing childbirth in French West Africa', in J. Allman, S. Geiger and N. Musisi (eds), *Women in African colonial histories* (Bloomington: Indiana University Press, 2002), pp. 71-91; Hunt, *A colonial lexicon*; W. T. Kalusa, 'Language, medical auxiliaries, and the reinterpretation of missionary medicine in colonial Mwinilunga, Zambia, 1922-1951', *The Journal of Eastern African Studies*, 1: 1 (2007), pp. 57-78.
31 Horwitz, *Baragwanath Hospital*, pp. 119-60.

32 Report of the Secretary for Health for the year ending 31 December 1966.
33 See last section of Chapter 2. See also, Masakure, 'One of the most serious problems confronting us at present', pp. 109–31.
34 See last section of Chapter 2. See also, Masakure, 'One of the most serious problems', and for South Africa see for example Burns, 'A man is a clumsy thing who does not know how to handle a sick person'.
35 National Archives of Zimbabwe (NAZ) S 2177/3/3 Salisbury Hospital: Correspondence: 1928-1948; S 119/1 Report of the Committee to review conditions of services for nurses in government employment, 1944.
36 NAZ F 242/SM/300/26 Southern Rhodesian Nurses Association.
37 NAZ ZBP 4/1/1 National Health Services Commission Report.
38 F. Cooper and A. L. Stoler, *Tensions of empire: Colonial cultures in a bourgeoisie World* (Berkeley: University of California Press, 1997), p. 17.
39 NAZ ZBP 2/1/3 National Health Services Commission. Oral evidence by B. Mnyanda, African representative to the National Health Services Commission, dated 18 September 1945 and NAZ ZBP 2/1/3, The Bulawayo Bantu Community Association, Memorandum to the National Health Services Commission, (n.d.).
40 A. L. Stoller quoted in A. F. Isaacman and B. Isaacman, *Dams, displacement, and the delusion of development* (Pietermaritzburg: University of Natal Press, 2013), p. 20.
41 See B. Raftopoulos, 'The crisis in Zimbabwe, 1998-2008', in B. Raftopoulos and A. Mlambo (eds), *Becoming Zimbabwe: A history from the pre-colonial period to 2008* (Harare: Weaver Press, 2009), pp. 201-32.
42 M. Echenberg, *Africa in the time of cholera: A history of pandemic from 1815 to the present* (Cambridge: Cambridge University Press, 2011), pp. 163-73 and C. Masakure, 'The politicisation of health in Zimbabwe: The case of the cholera epidemic, August 2008 – March 2009', *New Contree*, 80 (2018), pp. 65-88.
43 Interview: Mrs Estella Dhlamini, Harare, 22 August 2008.
44 Interview: Mrs Phaina Nyanhanda, Harare, 15 August 2007. Interview by P. Mukwambo.
45 Interview: Mrs Nomsa Makoni, Chitungwiza, 20 April 2009.
46 *The African Weekly,* 5 July 1961.
47 Interview: Mrs Nomsa Makoni, Chitungwiza, 20 April 2009.
48 Interview: Ms Tsitsi Chinamasa, Old Mutare Mission, 28 May 2009.
49 Interview: Mrs Laiza Shumba, Mabelreign Harare, 26 October 2008.
50 M. Trouillot, *Silencing the past: Power and the production of history* (Boston, MA: Beacon Press, 1995), p. 15.
51 Interview: Mrs Estella Dhlamini, Harare, 22 August 2008.
52 Physicians for Human Rights, *Health in ruins: A man-made disaster in Zimbabwe* (Cambridge, MA: Physicians for Human Rights, 2008/9), p. vi.

53 See T. Giles-Vernick, 'Oral histories as methods and sources', in E. Perecman and S. R. Curran, *Handbook for Social Science field research: Essays and bibliographic sources on research design and methods* (Thousand Oaks, CA: Sage Publications, 2006) pp. 85–95.
54 This is a popular derogatory term used on daily basis to refer to War Veterans and ZANU PF who have used war experiences to legitimise their monopoly over political space.
55 Interview: Mrs Nomsa Makoni, Chitungwiza, 20 April 2009.
56 Interview: Mrs Laiza Shumba, Mabelreign Harare, 26 October 2008.

2

The experiences of the pioneer generation of nurses, c. 1900–49

The introduction of the hospital system and by extension biomedicine had a significant impact on Africans in Southern Rhodesia. Introduced with different intentions by missionaries, the government and mining companies, biomedicine and the hospital system made a new therapeutic system available to Africans. Africans' responses to the presence of the new healing system varied across time and space. However, by the 1950s, Africans accessed hospitals in higher numbers than before. Although missionaries, the government and mining companies attracted medical and nursing personnel from abroad, the hospital system relied on a host of African assistants – in various capacities – to provide medical and nursing services to their fellow Africans.

I will sketch the histories of the women and men who embraced the opportunities offered by missionaries and the state to serve their people. Focusing on a broad spectrum of 'Native Assistants' – consisting of female and male nursing assistants, medical assistants and nursing orderlies – this chapter examines the various roles that women and men played in the provision of medical services to Africans. Following in the footsteps of L. Bryder's work on indigenous nurses in New Zealand, this is not a celebratory account of nurses 'rescuing "natives" fighting ignorance and superstition', nor is it an account of nurses being agents of missionaries or the colonial state.[1] Rather, the history of medical auxiliaries allows us to appreciate the importance of a cohort of women and men who not only took up hospital work to improve themselves, but also played an important role in the provision of biomedical services to their fellow Africans. Nursing orderly Kufa Mutoro underscored the role these medical auxiliaries undertook when he reflected that 'during the early years, it was difficult. These men and women made it happen. They paved the way for us, and we appreciate how they set the foundation for future hospital workers.'[2] An examination of their work must consider the disease environment in which the nursing orderlies and assistants worked. Like their counterparts in other parts of Africa, the medical auxiliaries inherited the diseased world of the late nineteenth century. They also experienced new medical conditions due to the expansion of the colonial economy, just as they encountered new diseases such as influenza.

While missionaries in-house trained the medical auxiliaries, the late 1920s saw a shift in the training of nurses at mission stations in Southern Rhodesia. Therefore, I will also examine the early efforts by missionaries to provide nurse-training institutions for Africans. Supported by a government medical grant, mission-trained nurses constituted the next generation of nursing personnel to work in mission hospitals in Southern Rhodesia. However, while the government supported missionaries with a medical grant, it did not formally recognise the mission nurses as 'trained'. Obsessed with standards, the colonial government also began to train medical orderlies in 1935. By this time, the government had started the transformation of medical service provision in rural areas. In addition to examining their training and briefly sketching their experiences, I discuss the training and role of what the government called the Advanced Male Native Nursing Orderlies. The government expected male nursing orderlies to be the bastion of biomedicine in government clinics in African areas. Although the government focused on rural areas in the 1930s and 1940s, medical service provision in urban areas was also in crisis. Specifically, African hospitals in urban areas experienced a shortage of nursing personnel. For African urban areas, the government wanted another type of nursing personnel: the State Registered Nurse (SRN), also referred to as the qualified nurse. There were debates in the mid-1940s that emphasised the need for African SRNs. From these debates, authorities reached a consensus on the need for the government to train African female SRNs, in the process marginalising the possibility of having male SRNs. These discussions set the foundations for new African nursing services dominated by African women in the post-1950 period.

The world of early medical auxiliaries

Until colonial medical authorities restructured the government rural clinic system in the 1930s,[3] the provision of medical services to Africans in rural areas was the responsibility of missionaries.[4] Missionaries, according to D. Hardiman, saw themselves as 'providing a ray of hope in a surrounding sea of darkness'.[5] Within the world of missionary activities, the field of healing attracted converts. Following in the footsteps of David Livingstone, missionaries who came to Southern Rhodesia emphasised the introduction of medical services to Africans as a key component of their missionary work. Megan Vaughan argued that, for many a missionary, mission medicine 'was part of a programme of social and moral engineering through which "Africa" would be saved'.[6] Four years into colonial rule, Dr John Helm, based at Morgenster Mission under the Dutch Reformed Church, became the leading figure in the provision of medical services to Africans within the vicinity of the mission station, while Dr W. L. Thompson of the American Board Mission provided medicine in the south-eastern parts of the country.[7] The Anglican Mission in the Umtali district began proselytising among Africans in the eastern districts with a medical mission,[8] while the Methodist Episcopal Church at Old Umtali Mission had Dr Samuel Gurney as the leading medical missionary by 1903.[9] The Catholic Jesuits at Bulawayo and the London Missionary Society at Inyati Mission and Hope Fountain Mission saw fit to commence their missionary work with a trained medical expert.[10] By the end of the first decade of the twentieth century, every mission station situated across the length and breadth of the colony had at least a dispensary or a makeshift hospital. For example, in 1903, the 'hospital' at Old Umtali consisted of an old ant-eaten building; after the First World War, it was a small brick building of poorly lit rooms. Each of the rooms had a window 'large enough to admit some rays of light but not admitting light enough to permit proper examination of patients much less the proper treatment'.[11] It was, according to Dr Samuel Gurney, 'unsuited for the work required'.[12]

The success of missionary work in general and missionary medical work in particular, relied on the availability of funds and Africans' responses. Furthermore, the functioning of medical missions also depended on the presence of a host of African medical assistants – the pioneer generation of medical auxiliaries and nurses. In the early days, knowledge of the English language was an underlying qualification for one to be recruited for hospital work. For example, converts who were pastors/teachers also acted as medical assistants. Converts such as C. Yafele, M. Kanogoiwa, Muti M. Sikobela and Tizora M. Neves were not only important in the spreading of missionary work for the Methodist Episcopal Church in the eastern districts of the country, they also played a significant role in helping '[cure] a large number of Natives, who have come, and sent to us imploring aid'.[13] Tizora M. Neves 'had a good knowledge of the Native character and his judgement and character have been of much benefit to us'.[14] Because of him and other assistants, many Africans not only sought medical assistance but 'were turning to the Great Physician for the healing of their souls'.[15] While Neves and others were not former patients but converts who took advantage of the situation, others, who turned to medical work, were former patients of missionary doctors or took up the job when missionaries introduced biomedical services in areas they inhabited.[16] Vaughan noted that a lengthy stay in hospital was some form of a rite of passage as it provided the patient with the spiritual and medical training for the job.[17] Nursing orderly Jonathan Manyoka's case is emblematical.[18] A leprosy patient, Jonathan Manyoka was born in 1907. His mother and brother died from leprosy. On 19 August 1925, he felt itching and saw marks on his body. Like most Africans during that time, he visited several indigenous doctors, the *n'angas*, who confirmed leprosy. According to Manyoka, the *n'angas* 'tried various treatments but without success'.[19] On the advice of Rev. T. Ferrel, he went to Nyadiri Mission near Mtoko to consult Dr Montgomery who also confirmed his leprosy case. He started his treatment in 1926. In the same year, Dr Montgomery offered him the position of nursing orderly at the leprosarium. His main tasks included giving 'quinine to others' and, in the afternoon, to 'teach the young leprosy patients'.[20] Jonathan Manyoka was paid 5 shillings a month for the job, and by the time he was discharged in 1929, Dr Montgomery increased his wage to £2 a month.[21] After his discharge, Manyoka stayed at the leprosarium to nurse and teach until 1950.

The mission records mention the majority of the early assistants in passing, but others were celebrated for a long time. One such man was Job Tsiga. In the 1960s, the Methodist Episcopal Church bulletin dedicated an entire page to his medical work.[22] Like many of his generation, he lacked formal education. Tsiga worked with Gurney, first at Old Umtali Mission and later at Mrewa Mission. The records consulted are silent on his date of birth. However, he was a convert by 1903 when Gurney became a medical missionary at Old Umtali Mission. In his later days, Tsiga was known for his dental work at Mrewa Mission.[23] In the 1960s, the Methodist members celebrated Tsiga for assisting one of the surgical operations that transformed the Methodist Church's fortunes at the end of the first decade of the twentieth century. During the harvest season in Mrewa district in 1909, an infuriated bull tossed into the air a young woman named Chemhunga. She and her friends were playing near a hut:

> We saw a large bull coming from a distance towards us … Then the bull came towards us with its head down, bellowing and we all ran for a place of safety. I did not escape he came directly at me. His sharp horn went through my side and he threw me up in the air. He picked me up on the horns when I came down and he threw me up in the air a second time.[24]

Her mother and brother washed her wound, pushed the intestines in, sewed the wound with a bark string, and tied a white cloth over it. The use of the bark string for wounds was an indigenous practice. Her brother carried her for about five kilometres to the government office. The government officer sent for Gurney and Job Tsiga. With Tsiga's assistance, Gurney cleaned the intestines and sewed the torn side.[25] The healing process took several months. Chemhunga's incident became a turning point in Tsiga and Gurney's medical work in Mrewa. After the operation as Tsiga narrated, 'I was asked to start a school … this is where Mrewa Mission stands'.[26] Tsiga was very clear on the overall impact of the surgical operation. Not only did Chemhunga's people convert to Christianity, but the operation also opened up space for the acceptance of their medical work by the inhabitants of the area.

Job Tsiga was one of the many medical auxiliaries who took up the opportunity made available by missionaries to provide biomedical services to their fellow Africans. They were the pacesetters to the later generation of nurses and medical auxiliaries who practised their trade across the length and breadth of Rhodesia. Early auxiliaries in the mould of Tsiga operated in tough circumstances, given the wide range of diseases they encountered. Using the case of East Africa, John Iliffe described the late ninetieth and early twentieth centuries as the 'age of agony'.[27] The same description can be applied to Rhodesia. The leading causes of mortality amongst Africans in Rhodesia in the first decade of the twentieth century were malaria, pneumonia, typhoid and dysentery.[28] In addition, the constant movement of people spread infectious diseases such as smallpox, which auxiliaries frequently encountered. Smallpox was prevalent in 1903, 1904, 1913 and 1921, which led the government to vaccinate approximately 90,000 Africans.

Furthermore, the spread of venereal disease in the first half of the twentieth century transformed the disease landscape in African areas where medical auxiliaries worked. From the 1900s onwards, reports from the Medical Officer of Health carried a section focusing on venereal diseases among Africans, with syphilis being the most prevalent.[29] Data indicate close connections between the high incidence of venereal diseases and the establishment of mines and towns that depended on African labour migration. The impoverished socio-economic environment of mines and towns, along with gender disparities and commercialised sex, predisposed men and women to enter short-lived relations conducive for the spread of venereal diseases. By the beginning of the First World War, mine owners were screening Africans for sexually transmitted diseases. During the wartime period, concerns about the 'venereal infected Natives' were raised and discussions on the need to protect Europeans from Africans infected with venereal diseases took place.[30] In 1917, authorities extended the examinations to points of entry. In 1918, Umtali Town Council became the first local council in Rhodesia to request permission to screen for venereal diseases Africans entering the town seeking employment.[31] By the early 1920s, Gurney, who worked with Tsiga, underscored that 'Venereal diseases are also constantly with us … the country is full with [sic] it.'[32] A significant number of Africans suffering from venereal diseases turned to missionary doctors and their assistants for treatment.

One should not underestimate the impact of the mining sector in transforming the disease environment in early twentieth-century

Rhodesia. Similar to what happened in other parts of southern Africa, colonial mining introduced occupational health problems for African workers. Chief among these were lung diseases such as tuberculosis and silicosis.[33] Furthermore, inadequate food supplies and poor living and working conditions severely affected African miners' health. Charles van Onselen noted that during the early years of the mining industry, dysentery and diarrhoea were common afflictions.[34] In 1911, the government brought into force new regulations dealing with African mine workers' sanitation and health. The regulations compelled mining companies to improve diet and ensured better working and living conditions for miners.[35] While mining companies accepted the need to enforce better standards of living and improved diet, the implementation was problematic. For example, the scurvy problems among miners continued. The 1914 Public Health Report noted that 'shortages, especially of beans and fresh vegetables, were reported from many districts as many of the articles were difficult to acquire'.[36] Such shortages adversely affected the health of many miners.

Ian Phimister demonstrated that mining companies sacrificed African workers' health at the altar of economic profits.[37] Furthermore, a guaranteed supply of cheap labour meant that 'there was no need for large-scale expenditure on medical care'.[38] Quality of medical care at the mines was thus inadequate. The unpopularity of mining hospitals amongst African miners is not surprising. Workers referred to the hospitals as *Imba Nema* – the 'Black House'.[39] At times, mining companies fenced these rudimentary hospitals to keep patients within the hospitals' premises and occasionally used 'Hospital Police Boys' to stop patients from leaving the hospitals.[40] African workers instead preferred treatment at mission stations. As the Board of Foreign Missions of the Methodist Episcopal Church wrote, 'The increase in mine workers has also meant an increase in work among those as yet outside the Church and an opportunity to show the meaning of the love of our Lord ... When accidents occur in the mines the sufferers look to the Mission for help'.[41] Hence, for those medical missions located near mining centres, the African mine worker and the medical problems he brought from the mines became the responsibility of mission doctors and their African assistants.

The occurrence of new diseases also shaped the world of medical auxiliaries. The influenza epidemic immediately comes to mind.[42]

Known as *vera* or *shuramatongo* by the locals, influenza made its first appearance in October 1918. An estimated 19,603 Africans and 303 whites died because of the epidemic in Rhodesia.[43] Influenza spread via the lines of communication, especially the railway, where the first reported cases appeared in Bulawayo among railway workers.[44] Following the railway line, it spread from Bulawayo to Que Que, Umvuma and to the capital, Salisbury, 'saturating most other areas that had highly concentrated population'.[45] In their efforts to contain the epidemic, authorities initially focused on urban centres. The government left rural areas, including mines, farms and African reserves, to fend for themselves.[46] According to Simmons, many Africans quickly left European areas such as towns and mines where influenza was prevalent, further spreading the disease to rural hinterlands.[47] For example, the Native Commissioner of Umtali noted that at Penhalonga mine, 'panic set in amongst the Natives at labour centres there, many of the Natives deserted and unfortunately, assisted in spreading the disease which practically visited all kraals (villages) in the district'.[48] The government deployed patrols to gather those who were fleeing.[49] Missionaries and their assistants also played a role in trying to control the movement of those suffering from influenza. Herbert Dzvairo, whose younger brothers died from influenza, stated that 'I was only saved by the fact that missionaries refused to let me go away. Had I tried (as some others did) to go away home, I would have died as others did.'[50] In addition, at mission stations, as Herbert Dzvairo continued, 'we were given some medicine which we drank and gurgled and also we had some medicines which we massaged on our arms so that blood vessels work freely'.[51] Considering the relative shortage of doctors and nurses when the epidemic broke out,[52] there is no doubt that Africans, some of them not trained in biomedical practices, played a central role in containing the disease. During the time of the epidemic, government officials 'used to send policemen with medicines into villages'.[53] In the Umtali district, one Frank Thompson, a visitor from Johannesburg, set up an isolation camp and hospital and supervised 'Cape boys and Native Assistants' who did 'most valuable work amongst Native patients'[54] (Figure 2.1). Within the same Umtali district, Fr Baker of the Church of England, 'assisted by 2 Native teachers, 6 adult Natives, and 6 youths,'[55] opened a hospital and a dispensary on the farm Lynnefield and from there

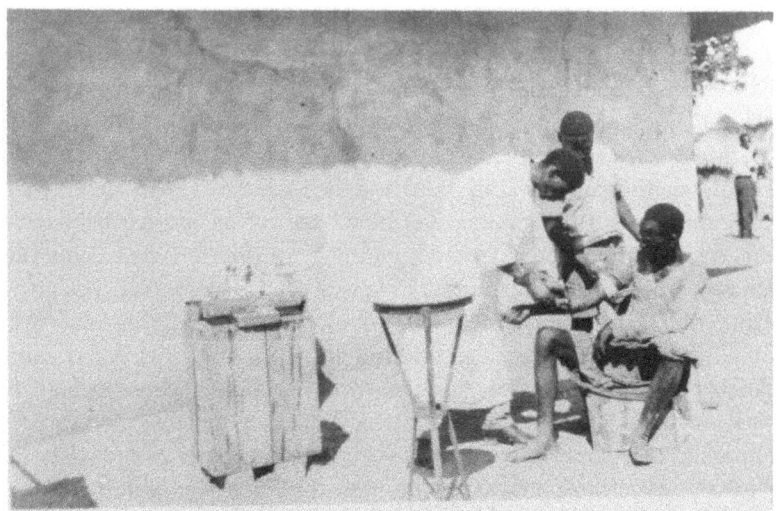

Figure 2.1 An early mission station clinic (courtesy National Archives of Zimbabwe)

distributed food and medicines, and directed 'his Native staff' in dispensing medicine within a radius of ten miles of the farm.[56] In the Melsetter district, one Roberts, a layman of the Methodist Episcopal Church, with the assistance of Africans, carried out inoculations near Mutambara Mission and within the radius of the mission.[57] The Native Commissioner of Salisbury underscored the work done by Africans during the epidemic when he stated that 'The Native messengers attached to this office did very good work.'[58] Like in East Africa, the influenza epidemic enlarged African subordinates' responsibilities.[59]

By the second decade of the twentieth century, African medical auxiliaries had established themselves as key components of the regime of care provided by mission stations. They had more responsibilities in the provision of medical care to Africans with little supervision from European hospital personnel, doctors and nurses alike. Medical auxiliaries were obliged to provide medical services to the converted who stayed far from mission stations. For example, some of the medical assistants at Old Umtali travelled from village to village, providing first-aid work. Although this was in line with African ideas of healing – where at times the *n'anga* (traditional healer) visited the patient to administer medicine – the missionaries encouraged this custom due to the unavailability of resources, the problem of distance, and, of course, as a way of proselytising. In her 1926 report, a white nurse at Old Umtali Mission, E. Bjorklund, not only highlighted the problem of 'pernicious malaria' in the area but also praised one of the medical assistants for his 'great talent in the care of the sick'.[60] According to Bjorklund, David Sakutomba 'has been walking from kraal to kraal (village to village) with a first aid box doing first aid work and preaching the gospel. This work has been much appreciated by our native friends, and many in this way have been brought under the influence of the word of God'.[61] By the 1920s, therefore, the medical auxiliaries had demonstrated their abilities. They were vital to the mission hospital. Even when this was the case, missionaries in the late 1920s began pushing for the formal training of mainly female nurses. In the process, they introduced another form of medical auxiliary work within the missionary regime of care as discussed below.

Mission nurses from the late 1920s to the 1940s

The 1920s saw a gradual transformation in the relationship between the government and medical missions and, by extension, the nursing profession among Africans in Rhodesia. Up to the early 1920s, missionaries relied solely on congregants abroad, in the mother churches in Europe and the United States, for the upkeep of medical missions.[62] Such contributions began to decline in the 1920s, which coincided with the call for the improvement of lives in rural areas. Influenced by the Christian missionary improvement ideology,[63] the call for improvement aimed at a greater increase in missionary work amongst Africans. In matters related to African health, missionaries requested government medical aid. They called on the government to provide more support for the provision of drugs and dressings or for the grants to cover such costs.[64] In 1926, a letter by Sr Elaine M. Lloyd based at St Faith Mission near Rusapi town underscored the lack of funding at mission stations by the mid-1920s:

> In our conversation, you [the Medical Director] said that probably the Government would be willing to assist if the work were already started. The annual expenditure of the Mission on drugs has been about £50 each for several years. This is practically spent on drugs, as for dressings we use

old material and our own cotton in place of 'cotton wool' ... All inpatients bring their own food[65]

St Faith Mission was not alone. Rev. C. A. Bowen, based at Dadaya Mission in Shabani, did not beat about the bush when he stated, 'we could use many more medicines if one had some extra assistance'.[66] In 1929, another missionary, H. W. Keynes of the Methodist Church wrote to the Native Department requesting aid:

> Would it be possible for you to arrange to let me have a small supply of medicines or bandages etc. for the use of the Natives around here? Since Mrs Keynes has been here, the Natives have been continuously coming for treatment of all descriptions. We have been giving medicines and dressing for months free, but we find we cannot continue doing so.[67]

The Southern Rhodesian Missionary Conference (SRMC), an umbrella organisation representing missionaries, was also seeking help from the government during the same time individual missionaries were. The SRMC urged the government to take full responsibility for Africans' healthcare in rural areas. The government, on the other hand, underscored the need for properly trained nursing and other auxiliary personnel as a condition for providing funding to medical missions. The Medical Director at that time, Dr Andrew Fleming, considered the training of medical auxiliaries, such as that of Tsiga or Sakutomba, as basic. Because of the nature of their training, he did not expect them to be at the forefront of providing services to their fellow Africans.[68] In fact, in the mid-1920s, Fleming took a random tour of mission stations. After visiting missions and mission schools 'in order to find exactly what was being taught in practical hygiene, maternity and childcare, he came to the conclusion that the results were not commensurate with the money and labour spent on them'.[69] He considered the efforts by missionaries a hopeless task. It was, therefore, the government's responsibility, as Fleming reasoned, to fund programmes to train African medical auxiliaries.

On 27 June 1927, the government introduced one of the 'most significant and progressive health measures'[70] – the legalisation of the payment of medical grants to medical missions by the Colonial Secretary, under government notice No. 335 of 1927. The government notice stipulated that medical grant recipients should employ 'qualified medical missionaries and certified nurses engaged in *bona fide* medical mission work in Native Reserves'.[71] At the same time, the government took responsibility for the payment of medical missionaries' and nurses' salaries.[72] The government also committed to pay for the purchase of drugs and dressings, including the upkeep of outdoor dispensaries.[73] The 1927 Government Notice thus set in motion the close relationship between the government and medical missions towards the provision of medical services to Africans in rural areas. As the Government Notice indicated, 'In respect of every approved medical mission station, the Government will contribute one half of the costs of all drugs, dressings and applications used, whether in dispensaries or outdoor relief, but no such contribution should exceed the sum of £100 ... in any year for any mission station.'[74]

The Government Notice also introduced a significant shift towards the training of African medical auxiliaries and nursing assistants. The government awarded a grant of £3 per bed per annum to each mission station for the upkeep of the mission hospital and guaranteed further finance to be used 'towards the establishment of training schools for Native probationer nurses, male and female'.[75] Unlike the earlier generation of medical auxiliaries, acceptance into nursing school depended on one having met 'an educational standard equivalent to European Standard IV',[76] an equivalent of six years of primary education.[77] For Africans in Rhodesia during the 1920s and 1930s, Standard IV was, without doubt, one of the highest educational achievements.[78]

Furthermore, the Government Notice laid down the minimum age of entrance into nursing school as well as the maximum time for training nurses. The minimum entrance age for male nurse probationers was twenty years, and seventeen for females. Their training covered a minimum of three years.[79] At the end of the course, the nurse received a certificate endorsed by the Public Health Department. The award of the certificate was subject to the probationer nurse passing an examination evaluated by government appointees.[80] To ensure the selection of the right candidates, the government paid medical missions a grant of £12 per annum 'for each completed year of service in respect of each fully certified nurse (male/female) employed by the mission'.[81] Through the Government Notice of 1927, the government showed its commitment towards African health in rural areas and kick-started the gradual transformation of African nursing services in Southern Rhodesia, laying the foundation for future nursing programmes.

In March 1928, missionaries held their annual conference in the capital, Salisbury. They welcomed the government's initiative but wanted to lower the age of entrance into nursing school. To be specific, they argued that as long as the candidate met the required standards for training, male nurse trainees could enter at sixteen and young women at fifteen.[82] Missionaries also requested that, in the event that missionaries employed a non-European Qualified Nurse to train Africans, the government should guarantee their wages just as they did for European nurses.[83] Finally, missionaries suggested introducing a two-year programme to train African midwives.[84]

In response, Dr Andrew Fleming agreed to amend the minimum age of entrance and to pay the same grant for non-Europeans engaged in the training of African nurse probationers, provided the African trainer possessed the same qualifications as the European one.[85] In relation to the training of midwives, the authorities tapped into the prevailing ideas about women and birthing processes. According to Gelfand, Fleming 'shared the point of view possibly current among members of the profession of that time that parturition was a natural procedure and that its processes were well known to the African woman. Therefore, he saw no reason to demand an educational standard for teaching methods of midwifery to African women.'[86] The connections between women and birthing practices continued throughout the colonial period. However, from the 1940s onwards, as the transformation of hospitals continued, the state began imposing strict education qualifications for women to be trained as midwives.[87] In the meantime, through the Government Notice 543 of 10 August 1928, the government authorised the payment of medical grants for the training of nurses at medical missions and the establishment of 'training schools for African probationer nurses of either sex'.[88]

Michael Gelfand credits Waddilove Mission as the first station that formally trained African nurses under the tutorship of Sr Madge Dry.[89] Sr Dry arrived at Waddilove Mission in 1927. At Waddilove, 'the hospital' consisted of a veranda of a small house, and Sr Dry used the bedroom as the main ward. Initially, she did the nursing of patients by herself, but in 1928 she recruited the first cohort of probationer nurses. Esther Maketo, Barbara Ben, Dinah Mgugu and Lilian Tyeza,[90] were the first young African women recorded to have entered nurse training modelled along the training methods used in government hospitals to train European nurses. After they passed their first examination,[91] the examiner, Dr T. G. Burnette of Bulawayo Hospital wrote, 'The training of Native girls in Nursing should be given every encouragement and should prove of great benefit, not only in the women's wards of Native Hospitals but in kraals (villages) to which some of these girls will return.'[92] The examination was divided into two parts: the theoretical – and the practical aspects of nursing. The following year, Sr Dry recruited five more young women. According to Sr Dry, their practical work was outstanding. Also, while not carrying the same grades as the first cohort on the theoretical part of their examination, Sr Dry considered the grades satisfactory.[93]

Sr Dry modelled her training along the lines of other nurse training courses presented to European student nurses at government hospitals. The first year focused on general nursing and the second year students concentrated on medical and surgical nursing, while students continued with surgical nursing in the third year. Their first-year course included ward cleaning, bathing patients, spreading the beds, recording temperatures, pulse and respiration, feeding patients and preparing minor dressings. Besides being introduced to daily work within wards in the second year, the teaching included giving enemas, douches, making different kinds of bandages, padding splints and assisting with more complex dressings. Their third-year practical work emphasised patient dressings under supervision, giving medicines, using hypodermic syringes, urine testing and writing reports. The third year also included special midwifery classes.[94]

Other medical missionaries followed in Waddilove Mission's footsteps. In 1930, Mt Selinda and Morgenster missions began training African nurses. Mt Selinda, in the eastern district of the country, accepted applicants with Standard IV being the minimum entrance qualification for their three-year course. The first cohort had seven students.[95] Morgenster had a cohort of eight probationers. Dr Steyn's letter thirteen years after the first cohort entered nursing school captured the progress made:

> From the very opening of our hospital in 1930, we considered it essential that we not only treat the sick, but train African nurses as well, to assist in our own hospital or elsewhere … The last 5 or 6 years we have been giving certificates to 4 to 6 girls every year. The certificates were given after a 3-year

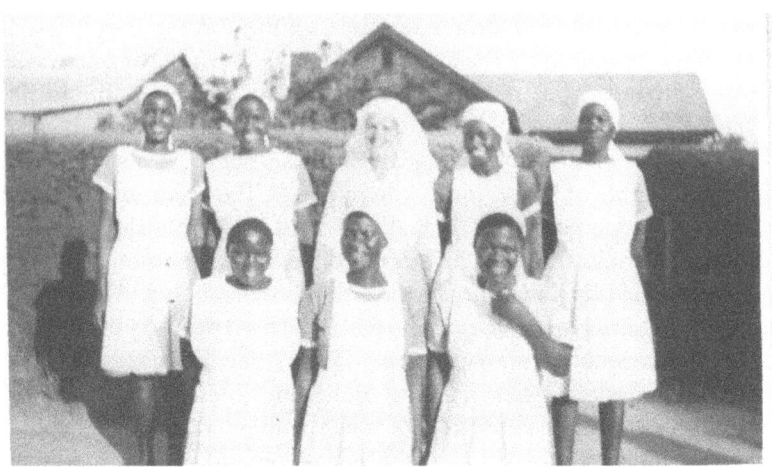

Figure 2.2 Sr Madge Dry with some of the nurses she trained (194-) [Date incomplete] (courtesy National Archives of Zimbabwe)

course in Nursing and Midwifery. Many of the girls have of course been married but quite a number are still nursing.[96]

For Dr Steyn, mission stations played an essential role in the training of nurses. Hence, the government had to continue supporting them. He continued,

> The possibility therefore, of mission hospitals training nurses, is not only practicable but I would venture to maintain that it would be a very short-sighted policy by those at the head of affairs if they fail to give every assistance possible to the mission and other hospitals to encourage them to train African nurses. With our new hospital of 60 beds, with brick huts for about another 120 patients and with an annual number of treatment of over 40 thousand, we hope to continue to the number of about 10 every year.[97]

Other mission stations, Howard, Mnene and Nyadiri followed Waddilove, Mt Selinda and Morgenster's examples. At Howard Mission, Sr Sloman began training probationer nurses in 1939. The first cohort had two nurse probationers, Rebecca Kudzai and Eva Sabangana, while the second cohort consisted of Grace Madenyika and Marty Moyo.[98] Mnene Mission, under the Church of Sweden, which operated in Matabeleland, started training in 1941 with sixteen students.[99] Nyadiri Mission began training nurse probationers in 1942, with Margaret Marange, Annie Gezi, Naomi Denga and Constance Chieza as the first students.[100] By 1943, at least seventy African female nurse students were in training at various mission stations across Rhodesia as shown in Table 2.1.

While some of these young women met the required education qualifications, at times missionaries ignored procedures to encourage young African women to enter nursing school. Sr Lorna Page, the first to train African nurses at Bonda Mission, commented on the quality of some of the young women at the beginning of the programme:

> At first, we had great difficulty in getting African girls for training – it was something unknown in that district, though mission hospitals existed in other parts of the country. The first girls were of a very low educational standard, local girls who were there only very temporarily (Standard I or II) … As time went on, we managed to get girls of higher educational standard.[101]

The cases of Monica Manawana, Miriam Majeke and Miriam Dhlembeu Moyo are emblematical. The three started their training at Bonda Mission in 1939. Manawana had experience in the hospital environment as she had worked at Rusapi Hospital, a government institution, for some years. Majeke worked for missionaries, most likely in the position of a nurse aide before she entered nurse training at Bonda Mission.[102] Dhlembeu Moyo wanted to work as a nanny since she did not meet the entrance level. When she arrived at

Table 2.1 The number of nurses in training at mission stations (1943)

	First year	Second year	Third year	Total
Bonda	3	2	4	9
Morgenster	7	7	3	17
Mnene	12	12	2	26
Mt Selinda	2	2	3	7
Nyadiri	2	5	-	7
Waddilove	-	1	3	4
Total	**26**	**29**	**15**	**70**

Source: ZBP2/1/2 Memorandum by the Federation of Women's Institutes of Southern Rhodesia to the National Health Services Inquiry Commission

Bonda Mission in September 1939, there was only one young woman (most likely Miriam Majeke) helping Sr Lorna Page in the hospital. Moyo later wrote that she was 'glad that Dr Taylor and Sister Lorna Page aimed for something else – that was for me to train as a nurse'.[103] She continued with her education while doing nursing: 'At that time I had to go to school and also start nursing. That means I was doing two things at the same time'.[104]

The experiences of student nurses differed from mission to mission. For Moyo and her cohort at Bonda, they woke up at 4 a.m. to fetch water from the well. In addition, they were expected to bathe patients, conduct general cleaning and cook.[105] A report from Mt Selinda highlighted the life of a student nurse in 1931 in this way:

> These students are all attending school from 6:30–10:00 save for two girls in the third-year course who give fulltime to their nurses' training. After 10:00, all are engaged in hospital work with the exception of one hour spent in supervised study. Saturday, they are on duty fulltime. Sunday, one boy [an orderly] and one girl are on duty all day, turnabout, the others off duty. During school holidays, each pupil is given one leave of two weeks per year. The question of giving two leaves [sic] of 2 weeks each year is under discussion. During the remainder of the holidays they are on duty at the hospital and dispensary.[106]

In reading the primary material, one gets a sense that although some of the nurses had not attained the required standards of education, the missionaries nevertheless produced well-rounded nurses. These nurses laid the foundation for the later generation of nurses who pursued State Registered Nursing in the post-1950 era. Yet, despite the students' training in most aspects of nursing, colonial medical authorities were hesitant to classify these women as 'fully trained nurses'. The cases of student nurses from Waddilove, the first mission to train nurses on a European model in government hospitals, comes to mind. Obsessed with standards and quality, the Medical Director claimed in 1932 that because there was no medical practitioner (doctor) attached to the mission and since the 'hospital' at Waddilove was small and thus did not treat a wide range of diseases, 'it was not considered that an efficient and comprehensive training could be given'.[107] It must be noted that the government gave different excuses in its refusal to recognise nurses trained at mission stations as 'fully trained nurses'. Such verdicts were frustrating for many missionary medical personnel, including Dr Steyn who observed, 'What we must insist on, however, is that there will be the same certificate for all African nurses whether trained in government, mission, mine or any other recognised hospital. I should also prefer the certificate to be given by the Medical Council as being a more representative body than even the Government.'[108] Steyn was writing in the 1940s, but in the 1930s, when missionaries were investing their time in training African nurses, the government commenced its training programme for government hospitals in rural areas. The nurse orderly programme, discussed in the next section, focused on the training of Advanced Native Male Nursing Orderlies. For officials, the government's programme was a panacea to the so-called problem of quality amongst the mission-trained nurses.

The Advanced Male Native Nursing Orderly

The training of the Advanced Male Native Nursing Orderly (nursing orderly) was closely linked to the government's formulation of a new medical scheme in African areas in the 1930s. Under the new medical scheme, the government had to establish a central hospital and sub-clinics in each district across the country. The Government Medical Officer (GMO) administered the everyday activities at the central hospital. The responsibility of running sub-clinics lay with African nursing orderlies. The GMO visited the sub-clinics on an occasional basis. The government set the plan in motion between 1931 and 1932. The Medical Director, Dr Robert A. Askins, who replaced Dr Fleming as the Medical Director in 1929, appointed Dr James Legate, a full-time medical officer to head the Mtoko medical centre.[109] A graduate of the London School of Tropical Medicine, Legate worked with an unnamed African medical assistant.[110] Askins also appointed Dr James Kennedy to head the Ndanga medical unit in 1932.[111] The government chose Mtoko and Ndanga due to the presence of a large African population in these districts. The two centres provided the basis for the provision of medical services in African areas in Southern Rhodesia. By 1936, thirty rural clinics across the country were either functioning or under construction.[112] By 1942, the inpatient accommodation at the main rural hospitals ranged from forty to 240 beds.

In the case of sub-clinics, the number of beds ranged between ten and forty. The GMO visited the sub-clinics as often as needed, ranging from twice a week to once a fortnight. The nursing orderlies in charge referred severe cases to the central hospital for treatment.[113]

Table 2.2 shows an increase in the number of sub-clinics as well as patients treated there over a period of ten years. The success of such a scheme rested on the government's ability to train enough medical and nursing personnel. While the GMO and European nursing personnel staffed the central hospital, the African staff provided the day-to-day nursing services. According to Gelfand, 'African men and women would be trained as orderlies and midwives to serve the central hospital and dispensary (sub-clinic)'.[114] Instead of relying on missionaries for training, the government with the help of the Medical Council of Rhodesia, trained the orderlies.[115] Dr Andrew Paton Martins, who took over the position of Medical Director in 1935, implemented Askins' vision of training medical orderlies. The *Government Gazette* of 18 June 1937 provided the regulations to train male orderlies.[116] Modelled along training programmes in the British colonies of Nyasaland and Kenya,[117] the programme set in motion the beginning of a government trained nursing orderly scheme and became the foundation of later African nursing programmes in Rhodesia. Nursing candidates should have attained Standard VI in order to qualify for training. Up to 1945, the government opened the course only to men,[118] but the same year, Bulawayo Hospital began to train women as well.[119] The first cohort of male orderlies at Salisbury Hospital consisted of Julius Gothosa, James Magole, William Titus Madeya and Robinson Tholana Mhlope. David Gunapira and

Table 2.2 A summary of government clinics and patients treated between 1936 and 1946

Year	Number of clinics	Inpatients treated	Outpatients treated
1936	21	11,422	22,704
1941	53	45,948	71,620
1946	73	71,620	245,138

Source: Compiled by the author from the Report of Public Health (1936, 1941 & 1946)

E. Myambe later joined them.[120] At Bulawayo, the cohort included Richard Musa, Simon Nguni, Howard Sibanda, Martin Maseko and Timothy Sidambe, who it seems moved to Salisbury.[121]

The preliminary examination in the first year consisted of anatomy and physiology, nursing, hygiene, admitting patients, bandaging, recording temperatures, charting and observing patients.[122] While it is not clear at what point in the first year they sat for the written examination and took the oral preliminary examination,[123] the examinations ascertained the suitability of the candidates to the nursing programme. Initial failure led to disqualification.[124] Over the three years of their training, nursing orderlies majored in medicine and surgery, medical and surgical nursing and advanced hygiene.[125] The authorities designed the advanced hygiene part of the course with the African village in mind. To be specific, the hygiene training focused on the planning of villages, identifying clean sources of water for drinking purposes, sanitary arrangements within the villages, disposal of household refuse, recognition of diseases and rudimentary treatment of ailments that affected Africans at the time.[126]

One of the challenges the programme faced in its early years centred on the availability of teaching staff. In a letter to the National Health Services Commission, a long-time administrator at Salisbury General Hospital, B. Gilbert, lamented that too few lecturers adversely affected the quality of teaching. Gilbert wrote:

> They have insufficient demonstrations and lectures and no teaching ward rounds ... The lectures and demonstrations are conducted by a Sister and a Government Medical Officer. Normally, the GMO, who has a multitude of other duties to perform, has little time for teaching, and one should remember that the giving of lectures entails the temporary loss of student orderlies from the ward or the loss of a Sister or GMO from their hospital duties.[127]

With such a situation, Gilbert reasoned that African nursing orderlies were 'scratching the surface of their medical education'.[128] As part of the solution, he suggested the use of senior orderlies as mentors to junior orderlies, guiding them in practical work and freeing up tutors to concentrate on other hospital work. Gilbert continued:

> In my opinion the best practical teaching, that is, in the wards would be obtained by the introduction into teaching hospitals of senior orderlies who have had experience of work outside clinics or head orderlies or whatever

you would like to call them. Their duties will be confined to certain wards, for example, Medical or Surgical; they should take all case histories, because of their ability to speak native tongue and to instruct the junior student orderlies who pass under their care year by year. The appointment should be sufficient enough to persuade the men to stay in their jobs for years.[129]

The government implemented the idea. Gelfand noted that 'of great help to the school was Mr Godfrey Muhango, a medical assistant, who joined the Salisbury Training School as an instructor'.[130] Muhango's name popped up in an interview with orderly Mutoro, who claimed that the earlier generation of auxiliaries who worked with Muhango and were likely trained by him, praised the man's sterling work.[131]

Once at rural clinic stations, the nursing orderly did a remarkable job in providing medical services to those needing help (Figure 2.3). In his reflection on the significance of nursing orderlies, reclassified as medical assistants in 1963, the Secretary for Health stressed the centrality of this category of hospital worker in rural areas. He wrote, 'He was never a type of inferior male nurse, but his training was designed for breadth rather than depth, as his role was to give timely treatment in minor diseases and recognise and refer the more serious conditions. Thus, his place was not in large central hospitals but rural ones, where in the same way as medical personnel, he provided a useful service.'[132]

Each sub-clinic had African medical orderlies as key staff and the GMO visited once or twice a week or every fortnight.[133] Considering the poor road conditions in rural areas and the difficulty of travelling during the wet season, the GMO sometimes took more than two weeks to visit. In such cases, clinics could not 'be supervised by a medical practitioner at regular and frequent intervals'.[134] On one occasion between 1939 and 1941, the GMO took over a year to visit the clinics in the Gutu District.[135] During the Second World War, visits to sub-clinics far from the main hospital were also likely intermittent. Glen Ncube observed that the spacing of visits by the GMO left orderlies in sole charge of rural clinics.[136] In such situations, nursing orderlies became de facto medical authorities in African areas, wielding medical authority and having relative autonomy. They diagnosed diseases, treated patients and were in charge of referrals. The disease environment had not, in fact, changed much; patients still contracted malaria, smallpox, bilharzia and venereal diseases.

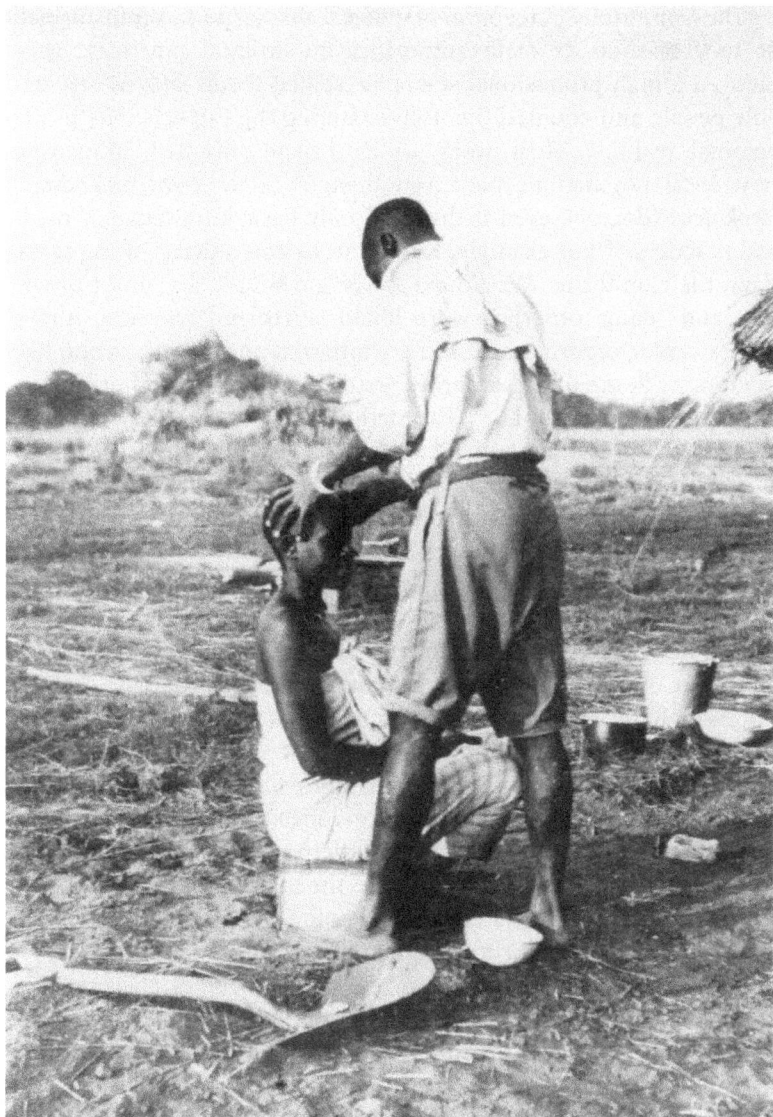

Figure 2.3 A medical orderly treating a patient (courtesy National Archives of Zimbabwe)

The community perception of medical auxiliaries was transformed as they became de facto authorities on hospital practices. They enjoyed a high professional status, presented themselves as respectable people and counted themselves among the top echelons in the colonial realm.[137] Their work, as Dr Legate reasoned, influenced how local populations perceived them.[138] Some were nicknamed *dhokotera* (doctor), even if they had only basic knowledge of medical practices.[139] For example, Kufa Mutoro noted that 'During those days, their uniforms were khaki shirts and shorts, for junior orderlies, and senior orderlies wore khaki shirts and trousers. Above that, a senior orderly possessed a white coat and a stethoscope like doctors … Some of the orderlies would even exhibit authority usually reserved for seniors.'[140] The stethoscope and a white coat were symbols of power and medical authority in Rhodesia, primarily preserved for white medical authority. By displaying such symbols in rural clinics in the 1930s and 1940s, medical auxiliaries not only appropriated the role usually reserved for trained medical personnel but also inserted themselves as pivotal in the smooth functioning of rural outposts. Such demonstrations were so common that one white female nurse at Mnene Mission complained to the National Health Services Commission, 'We do not want these male orderlies. They do not listen to us … they perceive themselves as medical doctors.'[141]

Government-trained nursing orderlies in rural areas also encountered responsibilities other than providing medical services at the sub-clinics. Like their predecessors, such as Job Tsiga and David Sakutomba, the missionary-trained orderlies and their counterparts in East Africa,[142] they were sent out to the surrounding villages, providing services to outdoor clinics, and in the process 'encouraging the sick to come to the clinic for treatment'[143] (Figure 2.4).

Besides encouraging more Africans to attend clinics, their responsibilities included being ambassadors for the new public health system. In 1938, the Medical Director noted that orderlies cured Africans in rural areas and gave 'lectures to Native villages on matters of hygiene and public health.'[144] The following year the Medical Director spoke about what he deemed to be the benefits of rural clinics and the presence of African nursing orderlies: 'the value of the outlying native clinic does not live purely in the curative aspect. These serve as a common nucleus for health propaganda throughout the remote

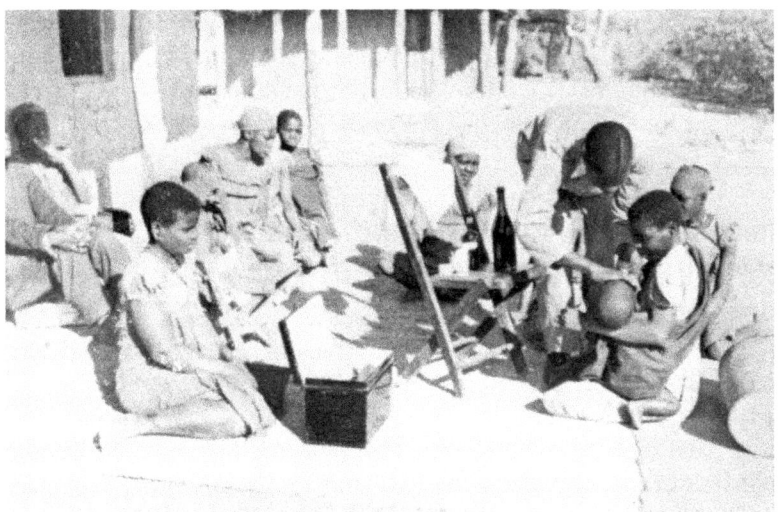

Figure 2.4 An outdoor African clinic (courtesy National Archives of Zimbabwe)

districts in which they are placed'.¹⁴⁵ Thus, while the nursing orderly demonstrated how good and efficient in curative practices he was, the government also transformed him into a preventative and propagandistic staff member.

The introduction of the Advanced Male Native Nursing Orderly training at Bulawayo and Salisbury set in motion the training of a host of other ancillary medical auxiliaries by the government in the 1940s. These included the training of female native nursing aides at Makumbi Hospital and native midwives at Umtali Hospital as the 1945 Public Health Report noted.¹⁴⁶ In the mid-1940s, the government arranged to train native women as mental nursing aides at Ingustheni Hospital in Bulawayo, and entered negotiations with the Royal Institute for the training and certification of native hygienists, the precursors of the Native Health Inspectorate.¹⁴⁷ Moreover, by the mid-1940s, the government commenced the training of African microscopists for clinical laboratory examinations.¹⁴⁸ The Umtali Native Midwives' Scheme was the first in which the government seriously considered women in more advanced roles within the broader nursing services. The introduction of the midwives' scheme coincided with the debates on the need for the government to train Africans as SRNs to work in government hospitals in urban areas. The debates led to the marginalisation of the training of male SRNs for government hospitals in Rhodesia until the mid-1960s, a subject discussed in the next section.

Debates over new African qualified nurses and the sidelining of male State Registered Nurses

While the government and missionaries were concentrating on African medical provisions in rural areas in the 1930s and 1940s, medical services to Africans in urban areas also needed urgent attention. Starting in the late 1930s, Rhodesia experienced a high rate of urbanisation. The situation that prevailed in the capital, Salisbury, illustrates this point. Between 1937 and 1949, Salisbury's estimated African population more than doubled, from 19,960 in 1937 to 59,358 in 1949. The population further rose by an estimated 90 per cent in the following five years, to 90,885.[149] Partly a result of the labour needs of the Rhodesian industries, the population increase in Salisbury in particular and other urban centres in general imposed burdens on nurses and hospitals. The case of one of Salisbury's townships, Harari, highlights this point. Between 1933 and 1943, patient visits at Salisbury's Harari Township Clinic increased from 2,608 to 36,668, and infant welfare clinic attendance rose from 466 to 6,850 between 1937 and 1943.[150] In general, accelerated urbanisation in the colony exposed the inability of nursing personnel to deal with the rapid changes taking place.

During the 1940s, government hospitals in urban areas experienced an insufficiency of trained staff and accommodation for African patients.[151] *The Bantu Mirror* of 14 August 1942 stated that at Salisbury General Hospital, 'There is not sufficient accommodation. There is great deal of congestion, and there are not sufficient nurses and sisters. We feel that something should be done about that. Sometimes the staff is obliged to discharge patients before they are completely cured.'[152] African patients were the victims of the staffing crisis, with female patients receiving less attention than men as well as limited access to facilities. Maternity cases were the worst affected. One of the leading members of the African middle class in the

1940s, B. J. Mnyanda, cited a case in Salisbury 'where a woman was unable to gain admission to the maternity clinic in the location and so she came to the Salisbury Hospital, but was refused admission'.[153] Although Mnyanda recounted only one incident, records show that such experiences were common, as white nurses struggled to cope with their increased workload. In 1944, one of Rhodesia's legislators, W. A Whittington, bemoaned that '[p]atients are turned away as was the case of a woman in labour. Both she and the child died.'[154] In 1945 Michael Gelfand exposed African patients' situation when he noted that 'The truth in my opinion, is that in the majority of the stations there is not enough time to treat the European and to give the Native better attention than is being done at the moment.'[155]

The training of African nurses to work in government institutions in urban areas would enable nursing and medical personnel to provide better attention to African patients. It must be noted that calls for the government to train Africans, especially women, began way before 1949. From the late 1930s onwards, pleas from all sections of Rhodesian society for the government to train African nurses in order to free white nurses to take care of white patients inundated the Medical Director's office. As far back as 1938 there were remonstrations from European patients at Salisbury General Hospital who objected to being nursed by white student nurses. They called upon the authorities either to speed up the training of more European nurses or to begin training African nurses to take care of African patients.[156] Two years later, the matron of the African section of Salisbury General Hospital complained bitterly about the extreme workload and implored the government to start training African SRNs as was already the case in South Africa.[157] In 1942, the senior Government Medical Officer at Bulawayo Hospital urged, '[t]he training of Bantu female nurses to work in the Native wards [is imperative] so as to set free the European personnel for European wards and thus lighten their burden'.[158] Such calls in Bulawayo coincided with Africans' demands for trained African nurses to work in African wards. In 1943, after a special meeting of the Bulawayo Bantu Community Association, a memorandum was sent to the head of the Municipal Department and the Clinic Committee of the Native Welfare Society indicating the need for African nurses in African wards.[159] In the memorandum, they strongly opposed:

> The principle of employing coloured nursing orderlies and midwives at the location clinic. The clinic was erected for the benefit of the African people and whenever feasible Africans deserve to be served by their own people, nurses and orderlies.[160]

Their calls were in line with what was taking place in Salisbury, where, by the mid-1940s, African nursing orderlies were employed at the Harari Township Clinic.[161] In 1945, the Coloured Services League wrote to the National Health Services Commission requesting the government to erect hospital wards for 'our own people', which would be staffed by coloured nurses.[162]

As much as practical reasons were behind the calls to have specific races concentrating on their own people and the shift in this regard – in Rhodesia as in South Africa – the drive towards training African SRNs for government hospitals had its origins in the general race relations of the colony. A history of race relations in Rhodesia indicates that from the 1920s onwards, the colony experienced a more rigid segregation policy.[163] According to P. R. Warhurst, besides the wish 'to preserve their (white) separate and superior position',[164] whites were motivated principally by the fear of the African, particularly the fear of the proximity between African men and white women. Ironically, it was within hospital settings that African men, as patients and workers, had close contact with white women – the nurses.[165] The proximity of African men to white women, either as patients or as workers (nursing orderlies) blurred the racial and gender boundaries that were central to the colonial order. The close association of African men to white nurses made the white community nervous. For example, in 1928 the *Rhodesian Weekly* alleged that African male convalescents were being cheeky to white nurses. After extensive investigations, the Secretary of General Salisbury Hospital claimed, 'no instance of the insolence of the kind described has been reported either to the Sister in Charge of the Native Hospital, the Acting Senior Government Medical Officer, or to myself'.[166] Although these allegations were false, anxieties over the proximity of African men to white women were always on the minds of white settlers. In South Africa, for example, scholars like Helen Sweet, Anne Digby, Catherine Burns and Shula Marks demonstrated how the racial fears of the proximity between white nurses and African males and the construction of the black men as threatening and uncivilised led to the debates on the need for African nurses.[167] Central to the anxieties was the issue of white female sexuality.[168] The most sensitive area of race relations, as Warhurst noted, was sex.[169] From 1902 to the mid-1930s, a series of panics, precipitated by the presumed sexual threat posed by black men to white women, swept across Rhodesia, in what scholars have termed the 'Black Peril' scares.[170] The white community in Rhodesia, as in South Africa, responded to the 'Black Peril' scares with efforts at establishing the boundaries of race, class and gender.[171] Such ideas, on the need to impose boundaries between white women and black men, were transferred to clinical spaces. Writing on South Africa, Shula Marks noted that from the 1920s onwards, it was becoming less acceptable for white female nurses to tend to black patients, male or female.[172] Such racist attitudes towards patient care[173] were replicated in Rhodesia. During the debate on hospitals in the Legislative Assembly, Captain W. A. Whittington spoke on behalf of many white Rhodesians when he said, 'I do not think that the present position is right, that Europeans should look after Natives.'[174] What he had in mind was not merely nursing care for Africans. To be specific, he referred to white nurses providing nursing care to African men. There were always anxieties about close contact between African male patients and white female nurses. These racial fears were inextricably intertwined with the construction of the idea of black men as 'threatening', of black men being profoundly 'unclean', and of black men being 'uncivilised'.[175] Of course, some Africans contested these views. No one brings the inconsistency into sharper focus than B. J. Mnyanda. In his critique of the policy of segregation, he wrote,

> It is incredible to believe that these very Europeans who are so eager to find fault with the Africans in the mass, sit down daily at breakfast, lunch and in the evening to sumptuous and delicious meals – all prepared entirely by African hands. Piccaninnies [African boys] and African nannies nurse and look after the welfare of young European children. In some cases, these servants look after the children while the mothers are away at work for the whole day.[176]

During the entire colonial period, African domestic servants, male and female alike, sustained white households. Within hospitals, white nursing staff and medical doctors in government and mission hospitals continued to take care of convalescent Africans. Even so, the racist views of people such as Captain W. A. Whittington played a significant role in influencing state policies.

Importantly, the envisaged training of African SRNs placed emphasis on female nurses. Yet men had always been employed as nurses at mines and in psychiatric hospitals.[177] In addition, as noted above, orderlies also practised every aspect of hospital work, including nursing. A veritable constellation of factors thus contributed to sidelining the training of male qualified nurses for general hospitals in the 1950s.[178] Besides official policy, which limited the training of qualified nurses to white women,[179] there was also the ongoing construction of gender roles linked to a timeworn Victorian ideology. Elizabeth Schmidt demonstrated the various ways such an ethos, as well as the sexual and gendered stereotypes imparted by missionaries and settlers, was inextricably intertwined with gendered discriminatory systems within African societies.[180] In nursing, this was done by emphasising the intimacy of nursing and the feminine qualities of the nursing profession. As Marks rightly noted, the dominance of women within professional nursing was 'related to both the gendered model of professional nursing imported from the metropole with its resonance in settler societies and the particularities of its racialised and gendered economy'.[181]

By the 1940s, chances for African males to train and work as qualified nurses in general hospitals were very slim.[182] For example, the Secretary of the General Salisbury Hospital, C. S. Mitchell, was against the idea of training male nurses because he had already worked with male orderlies, most of whom, in his opinion, 'neglect[ed] real nursing which can much more easily be developed from the natural temperament of the female. Women by their nature are more suitable than men for the job.'[183] In the same vein, Plof W. Nirdjesjo, a nurse at Mnene Mission, argued in 1945 that 'male orderlies are rougher than female orderlies'.[184] Such suggestions were central in influencing the policies that obstructed African men from pursuing nurse training. The first cohort of qualified African nursing students at Harare Hospital explicitly excluded men. Thus, on 1 September 1958, fifteen African student nurses began the journey of training as qualified nurses.[185] Trained at Harari and Impilo hospitals, they were the first cohort of African women to undertake the SRN programme in Rhodesia. These nurses, just as student teachers before them, represented the 'progress of African women', as the veteran nationalist, Edison Sithole, remarked.[186] The training of African nurses gradually transformed the Southern Rhodesian Nursing Services from being predominantly white to being more racially and ethnically diverse, including Africans, coloureds and Asians.

Conclusion

Like their counterparts who took up various aspects of medical practice in other parts of the continent at the end of the nineteenth century, the medical auxiliaries in Rhodesia were the pivot in the provision of medical services to Africans in rural areas. Broadly speaking, these medical auxiliaries included nurses, nursing assistants and nursing medical orderlies. These women and men took up employment opportunities made available by the introduction of biomedicine, and, in the process they were able to provide medical services to their fellow Africans. In the archives the majority of them are merely referred to as 'assistants'. A few were celebrated and mentioned by name. Yet, day and night, they toiled in hospitals, taking care of the sick and nursing the infirm. Working in the early colonial hospital had its challenges. The rudimentary nature of the hospital system moulded the world of these auxiliaries. The nature of diseases they encountered also shaped their world and their work. Besides, the transformation of the economy saw the spread of STDs and the 1918 influenza epidemic wreaked havoc in both black and white communities. As in other parts of Africa, African assistants played their fair share in fighting disease outbreaks.

Significant shifts also took place in the 1920s and 1930s concerning the training of nurses and orderlies for mission stations and government clinics. While the pioneer generation of nurses and medical auxiliaries were not formally trained, the grant offered to mission stations in 1927 would transform the nature of training. Following the South African example, mission stations began the formal training of African women as nurses. At the time that missionaries began training young women as nurses, the government was also envisioning its version of African medical auxiliaries. The Advanced Male Native Nursing Orderly, trained at Bulawayo and Salisbury, became the central figure in the provision of medical services within the rural clinic system in Rhodesia. They would play a central role in the expansion of medical services in rural areas. In most cases, these orderlies became de facto medical authorities in rural clinics. By the 1940s, Africans – nurses trained at mission stations and orderlies working at sub-clinics – had become instrumental in providing rural medical services.

While Africans had established themselves as key nursing personnel in rural clinics, the presence of Africans within urban hospitals and clinics that provided services to Africans residing in urban areas was limited. Hence, there were debates in the 1940s about the need to train another type of nurse to be in charge of African hospitals in urban areas – the State Registered Nurse (SRN). These debates set in motion the government's two-pronged strategy in transforming nursing services in Southern Rhodesia from the 1950s onwards. It offered bursaries to young women to train as nurses in South Africa and also to open up the training of SRNs to the non-European population of Rhodesia. In 1953, the government commenced the local training of coloureds and people of Asian origin as SRNs. Thus local training was extended to Africans in 1958 and by the 1960s, African SRNs were to become more visible in African hospitals. Even though the government focused on female SRNs, African women who entered the profession in the 1950s were important historical actors who, for various motives, chose to nurse as a preferred career option. What immediately follows is their story, putting into purview the motives for choosing nursing as a career option.

Notes

1 L. Bryder, '"They do what you wish; they like you the good nurse!": Colonialism and native health nursing in New Zealand, 1900–40', in Sweet and Hawkins (eds), *Colonial caring*, p. 85.
2 Interview: Mr Kufa Mutoro, Mutare, 12 August 2008.
3 It must be underscored that although the government was concerned about Africans' health up to the 1930s, its efforts at providing sustained health measures experienced mixed results. They focused mainly on specific diseases or epidemics, leaving the general provision of medical services to missionaries or mining companies. Even the government's early efforts at introducing dispensaries from 1912 onwards did not meet desired results due to the hesitant approach adopted by the Public Health Department. For more on this see

G. Ncube, 'The making of rural healthcare in colonial Zimbabwe: A history of the Ndanga Medical Unit, Fort Victoria, 1930-1960s' (PhD thesis, Department of Historical Studies, University of Cape Town, 2012), pp. 30-48.
4 M. Gelfand, *A service to the sick: A history of the health services for Africans in Southern Rhodesia.1890-1953* (Gwelo: Mambo Press, 1976), pp. 35-40.
5 D. Hardiman (ed.), 'Introduction', *Healing bodies, saving souls: Medical missions in Asia and Africa* (Amsterdam: Rodopi, 2006), p. 6.
6 M. Vaughan quoted in Hardiman (ed.), *Healing bodies, saving souls*, p. 6.
7 Gelfand, *A service to the sick*, p. 11.
8 Gelfand, *A service to the sick*, p. 11.
9 African University Archives: The Last Report of Dr Samuel Gurney to the Rhodesian Missionary Conference, United Methodist Church, 19-25 June 1923.
10 Gelfand, *A service to the sick*, p. 11.
11 Africa University Archives: The Last Report of Dr Samuel Gurney to the Rhodesian Missionary Conference, United Methodist Church, 19-25 June 1923.
12 Africa University Archives: The Last Report of Dr Samuel Gurney to the Rhodesian Missionary Conference, United Methodist Church, 19-25 June 1923.
13 Africa University Archives: Report of the Rhodesian Missionary Conference, United Methodist Church, 1909.
14 Africa University Archives: Report of the Rhodesian Missionary Conference, United Methodist Church, 1909.
15 Africa University Archives: Report of the Rhodesian Missionary Conference, United Methodist Church, 1909.
16 Vaughan, *Curing their ills*, p. 61.
17 Vaughan, *Curing their ills*, p. 61.
18 See D. A. W. Rittey, 'The story of a leprosy patient', *Central African Journal of Medicine*, 18: 11 (1972), pp. 230-2.
19 Jonathan Manyoka quoted in Rittey, 'The story of a leprosy patient', p. 231.
20 Jonathan Manyoka quoted in Rittey, 'The story of a leprosy patient', p. 231.
21 Jonathan Manyoka quoted in Rittey, 'The story of a leprosy patient', p. 231.
22 Africa University Archives, E. Sells, 'Medical Practice between "two worlds"': A woman tells how Dr Gurney put back her intestines', *Rhodesia – the Methodist Church – yesterday and today* (no date but likely published in the 1960s).
23 Africa University Archives, interview with Mrs Viola Chirimuuta, Mrehwa Mission, 3 May 2013. Interview by S. Machuma and recorded by G. Nera.
24 Africa University Archives, Sells, 'Medical practice between "two worlds"'.
25 Africa University Archives, Sells, 'Medical practice between "two worlds"'.
26 Africa University Archives, Job Tsiga quoted in Sells, 'Medical practice between "two worlds"'.
27 J. Illife, *East African doctors: A history of the modern profession* (Cambridge: Cambridge University Press, 1998), p. 9.
28 Government of Southern Rhodesia, Public Health Report 1911.

29 Gelfand, *A service to the sick*, p. 24.
30 L. Jackson, '"When in the white man's town": Zimbabwean women remember chibeura', in J. Allman, S. Geiger and N. Musisi (eds), *Women in African colonial histories* (Bloomington: Indiana University Press, 2002), pp. 191–215.
31 NAZ LG 104/48, Medical examination of natives, Memorandum by Medical Director.
32 Africa University Archives: The Last Report of Dr Samuel Gurney to the Rhodesian Missionary Conference, United Methodist Church, 19–25 June 1923.
33 For South Africa, see for example, R. Packard, *White plague, black labor: Tuberculosis and the political economy of health and disease in South Africa* (Berkeley: University of California Press. 1989) and J. McCulloch, *Asbestos blues: Labour, capital, physicians and the state in South Africa* (Oxford: James Currey, 2002).
34 C. Van Onselen, *Chibaro: African mine labour in Southern Rhodesia, 1900–1933* (London: Pluto Press, 1976), p. 51.
35 Government of Southern Rhodesia, Report of Public Health, 1911.
36 Government of Southern Rhodesia, Report of Public Health, 1914.
37 I. R. Phimister, 'African labour conditions and health in Southern Rhodesian mining industry, 1898–1953. Part IV; Hospitalisation and Conclusions', *Central African Journal of Medicine*, 22:12 (1976), pp. 244–9.
38 Van Onselen, *Chibaro*, p. 57.
39 Van Onselen, *Chibaro*, p. 59.
40 Van Onselen, *Chibaro*, p. 59.
41 Africa University Archives: Board of Foreign Missions, *On trek with Christ in Southern Africa*. Methodist Episcopal Church, (n.d.), p. 47.
42 For more on influenza in colonial Zimbabwe, see for example, I. R. Phimister, 'The "Spanish" influenza pandemic of 1918 and its impact on the Southern Rhodesian mining industry', *Central African Journal of Medicine*, 19: 7 (1973), pp. 143–8; T. O. Ranger, 'The influenza pandemic in Southern Rhodesia: A crisis of comprehension', in D. Arnold (ed.), *Imperial medicine and indigenous societies* (Manchester: Manchester University Press, 1988), pp. 172–88 and D. Simmons, 'Religion and medicine at the crossroads: A re-examination of the Southern Rhodesian influenza epidemic of 1918', *Journal of Southern African Studies*, 35: 1 (2009), pp. 29–44.
43 Simmons, 'Religion and medicine at the crossroads', p. 31.
44 During this time, Bulawayo was the headquarters of the Rhodesia Railways. For a general history of Bulawayo see T. O Ranger, *Bulawayo burning: A social history of a southern African town* (Harare: Weaver Press, 2010).
45 Simmons, 'Religion and medicine at the crossroads', p. 31.
46 Simmons, 'Religion and medicine at the crossroads', p. 31.
47 Simmons, 'Religion and medicine at the crossroads', p. 31.
48 NAZ N 9/1/21, Report of the Native Commissioner, Umtali District, 1918.

49 Simmons, 'Religion and medicine at the crossroads', p. 32.
50 Herbert Dzvairo quoted in Simmons, 'Religion and medicine at the crossroads', p. 33.
51 Herbert Dzvairo quoted in Simmons, 'Religion and medicine at the crossroads', p. 33.
52 Simmons, 'Religion and medicine at the crossroads', p. 31.
53 Mr Mhako quoted in Simmons, 'Religion and medicine at the crossroads', p. 33.
54 NAZ N 9/1/21, Report of the Native Commissioner, Umtali District, 1918.
55 NAZ N 9/1/21, Report of the Native Commissioner, Umtali District, 1918.
56 NAZ N 9/1/21, Report of the Native Commissioner, Umtali District, 1918.
57 NAZ N 9/1/21, Report of the Native Commissioner, Umtali District, 1918.
58 NAZ N 9/1/21, Report of the Native Commissioner, Umtali District, 1918.
59 Illife, *East African doctors*, p. 35.
60 Africa University Archives, E. E. Bjorklund, Report of Medical Work at Old Umtali, Rhodesia Mission Conference, Methodist Episcopal Church, November 1926.
61 Africa University Archives, E. E. Bjorklund, Report of Medical Work at Old Umtali, Rhodesia Mission Conference, Methodist Episcopal Church, November 1926.
62 NAZ S 1173/302, G. I. Phaepher, Antelope to J. C. Blackwell, 16 July 1925.
63 J. Alexander, J. McGregor and T. Ranger, *Violence and memory: One hundred years in the 'dark forests' of Matabeleland* (Harare: Weaver Press, 2000), p. 69.
64 Gelfand, *A service to the sick*, p. 112.
65 NAZ S 1173/302, E. M. Lloyd, St Faiths Mission, Rusape to Medical Director, 16 September 1926.
66 NAZ S 1173/302, C. A Bowen, Dadaya Mission, Shabani to Colonial Secretary, 11 October 1928.
67 NAZ S 1173/303, H. W Keynes, Hotsprings to O. Jackson, 26 September 1929.
68 Gelfand, *A service to the sick*, p. 114.
69 Gelfand, *A service to the sick*, p. 115.
70 Gelfand, *A service to the sick*, p. 116.
71 Government Notice No.335, 27 June 1927 (Government Printer: Salisbury, 1927).
72 Government Notice No.335, 27 June 1927 (Government Printer: Salisbury, 1927).
73 Government Notice No.335, 27 June 1927 (Government Printer: Salisbury, 1927).
74 Government Notice No.335, 27 June 1927 (Government Printer: Salisbury, 1927.
75 Government Notice No.335, 27 June 1927 (Government Printer: Salisbury, 1927).

76 Government Notice No.335, 27 June 1927 (Government Printer: Salisbury, 1927).
77 In South Africa in 1936 for example, the admission into both government and mission hospital training programmes required a Standard VII, while McCord required Standard IX. In 1942, in the Cape Province of South Africa, the admission requirements for both government and mission hospitals was a Standard VIII at Victoria Hospital and Lovedale Mission. See J. Parle and V. Noble, *The people's hospital: A history of McCord, Durban, 1890s-1970s* (Natal Society Foundation: Pietermaritzburg, 2018), p. 61.
78 For more on African education in colonial period, see for example, C. Summers, *Colonial lessons: Africans' education in Southern Rhodesia, 1918-1940* (Oxford: James Currey, 2002).
79 Government Notice No.335, 27 June 1927 (Government Printer: Salisbury, 1927).
80 Government Notice No.335, 27 June 1927 (Government Printer: Salisbury, 1927).
81 Government Notice No.335, 27 June 1927 (Government Printer: Salisbury, 1927).
82 NAZ S 1173/303, Resolution of the Southern Rhodesian Missionary Conference, Salisbury, 26–9 March 1928.
83 NAZ S 1173/303, Resolution of the Southern Rhodesian Missionary Conference, Salisbury, 26–9 March 1928.
84 NAZ S 1173/303, Resolution of the Southern Rhodesian Missionary Conference, Salisbury, 26–9 March 1928.
85 The medical authorities were strict when it came to certificates, insisting that they should confirm a training in general nursing. In 1934, the government refused to pay Nurse Joyce Pukwani's wages. Employed at Bonda Mission, Pukwani had trained in South Africa and according to the medical practitioner at Bonda Mission, Dr Lawrence, she had excellent references from South African authorities and was adept at her work. However, the medical authority refused to pay her wages because she had only furnished them with a midwifery certificate and not a general nursing certificate. See NAZ S 2014/6/21, Bonda Mission, letter from H. Lawrence to the Medical Director, 28 November 1933 and the reply letter from Medical Director to H. Lawrence, 8 February 1934.
86 Gelfand, *A service to the sick*, p. 118.
87 The Umtali African Midwives Government Training School opened in 1945 the general entrance was Standard VI. For more see Gelfand, *A service to the sick*, pp. 151–2.
88 Gelfand, *A service to the sick*, p. 118.
89 Gelfand, *A service to the sick*, p. 130.
90 NAZ S 2014/6/28, Waddilove Training Institution, Revd. John White to Medical Director, 15 June 1928.

91 NAZ S 2014/6/28, Waddilove Training Institution, T. G. Burnette, Report of Examination in Nursing, 7 December 1928.
92 NAZ S 2014/6/28, Waddilove Training Institution, T.G. Burnette, Report of Examination in Nursing, 7 December 1928.
93 NAZ S 2014/6/28, Waddilove Training Institution, Sister Madge Dry, Report on Waddilove Training Institution, 1930.
94 NAZ S 2014/6/28, Waddilove Training Institution, Sister Madge Dry, Report on Waddilove Training Institution, 1930.
95 NAZ S 2014, American Board Mission, Mt Selinda, Dr Lawrence to the Medical Director, 14 November 1930.
96 NAZ ZBP 2/1/3, National Health Services Commission, Dr M. H. Steyn, Morgenster Mission to J. Lenfesty, Gwelo Native Welfare Society, 26 April 1943.
97 NAZ ZBP 2/1/3, National Health Services Commission, Dr M. H. Steyn, Morgenster Mission to J. Lenfesty, Gwelo Native Welfare Society, 26 April 1943.
98 Gelfand, *A service to the sick*, p. 137.
99 NAZ S 2014/6/10, Mnene Report of the Medical Work carried out by the Church of Sweden Mission in Belingwe and Gwanda Districts in the year 1942.
100 NAZ S 2014/6/16, Report of Medical Work at Nyadiri, 1942.
101 Sr Lorna Page quoted in Gelfand, *A service to the sick*, p. 134.
102 Gelfand, *A service to the sick*, p. 132.
103 M. D. Moyo quoted in Gelfand, *A service to the sick*, p. 136.
104 M. D. Moyo quoted in Gelfand, *A service to the sick*, p. 136.
105 M. D. Moyo quoted in Gelfand, *A service to the sick*, p. 136.
106 NAZ S 2014/6/28, American Board Mission, Mt Selinda; 27 July 1925, 30 October 1947, Syllabus for Nurses' Training, Mt Selinda.
107 NAZ S 2014/6/28, Waddilove Training Institution, Medical Director to Principal, Waddilove Training Institution, 31 May 1932.
108 NAZ ZBP 2/1/3, National Health Services Commission, Dr M. H. Steyn, Morgenster Mission to J. Lenfesty, Gwelo Native Welfare Society, 26 April 1943.
109 Gelfand, *A service to the sick*, p. 123.
110 Gelfand, *A service to the sick*, p. 123.
111 For Ndanga, see G. Ncube, 'The making of rural healthcare in colonial Zimbabwe: A history of the Ndanga Medical Unit, Fort Victoria, 1930-1960s' (PhD thesis, Department of Historical Studies, University of Cape Town, 2012).
112 Government of Southern Rhodesia, Report of Public Health 1936.
113 Government of Southern Rhodesia, Report of Public Health, 1941-1945.
114 Gelfand, *A service to the sick*, p. 127.
115 *The Bantu Mirror*, 11 July 1936.
116 Gelfand, *A service to the sick*, p. 138.
117 *The Bantu Mirror*, 26 June 1937.

118 Gelfand, *A service to the sick*, p. 138.
119 Gelfand, *A service to the sick*, p. 127.
120 Gelfand, *A service to the sick*, p. 138.
121 Gelfand, *A service to the sick*, p. 141.
122 *The Bantu Mirror*, 24 December 1938.
123 *The Bantu Mirror*, 26 June 1937.
124 Interview: Mr Kufa Mutoro, Mutare, 12 August 2008.
125 *The Bantu Mirror*, 24 December 1938.
126 *The Bantu Mirror*, 24 December 1938.
127 NAZ ZBP 2/1/2, National Health Services Commission, B. Gilbert, The General Hospital Salisbury, letter to the NHSC, 1 March 1944.
128 NAZ ZBP 2/1/2, National Health Services Commission, B. Gilbert, The General Hospital Salisbury, letter to the NHSC, 1 March 1944.
129 NAZ ZBP 2/1/2, National Health Services Commission, B. Gilbert, The General Hospital Salisbury, letter to the NHSC, 1 March 1944.
130 Gelfand, *A service to the sick*, p. 139.
131 Interview: Mr Kufa Mutoro, Mutare, 12 August 2008.
132 Government of Southern Rhodesia, Report of Public Health 1964.
133 Government of Southern Rhodesia, Report of Public Health 1945.
134 Government of Southern Rhodesia, Report of Public Health 1946.
135 Ncube, 'The making of rural healthcare in colonial Zimbabwe', p. 178.
136 Ncube, 'The making of rural healthcare in colonial Zimbabwe', p. 178.
137 See A. Shutt's examination of a litigation case against defamation by one Ephraim who worked at a clinic in Wedza. A. Shutt, 'Litigating honor, defamation, and shame in Southern Rhodesia', *African Studies Review*, 61: 3 (2018), pp. 79–98.
138 Shutt, 'Litigating honor, defamation, and shame in Southern Rhodesia', pp. 79–98.
139 Interview: Mr Kufa Mutoro, Mutare, 12 August 2008.
140 Interview: Mr Kufa Mutoro, Mutare, 12 August 2008.
141 NAZ ZBP 2/1/3, National Health Services Commission, Plof. W. Nirdjesjo, Mnene Mission to the National Health Services Commission, 7 December 1945.
142 For East Africa, see Iliffe, *East African doctors*, p. 41.
143 Government of Southern Rhodesia, Report of Public Health 1938.
144 Government of Southern Rhodesia, Report of Public Health 1938.
145 Government of Southern Rhodesia, Report of Public Health 1939.
146 Government of Southern Rhodesia, Report of Public Health 1945.
147 Government of Southern Rhodesia, Report of Public Health 1945.
148 Government of Southern Rhodesia, Report of Public Health 1945.
149 See D. Johnson, *World War Two and the scramble for labor in colonial Zimbabwe, 1939–1948* (Harare: University of Zimbabwe Publications, 2000), p. 142.
150 NAZ LG 191/12/7/1, Native Welfare at the Location.

151 NAZ ZBP 1/2/4, National Health Services Commission, Dr R Mackenzie Honey, Oral evidence to the National Health Services Commission, 31 October 1945.
152 *The Bantu Mirror*, 14 August 1942.
153 NAZ ZBP 2/1/3, National Health Services Commission, B. Mnyanda, Oral evidence to the National Health Services Commission, 18 September 1945.
154 Captain W. A. Whittington, Legislative Assembly Debates, Volume 24, 1944, p. 871.
155 NAZ ZBP 2/1/3, National Health Services Commission, Michael Gelfand to the National Health Services Commission, 13 August 1945.
156 NAZ S 2177/3/3, Salisbury Hospital, Correspondence 1928–1940s, A. P. Martin, Memorandum on New Native Hospital, 20 April 1938.
157 For South Africa, see for example, Marks, *Divided sisterhood*.
158 NAZ S 2177/1/2, Nurses, General Correspondence, Senior Government Medical Officer, Memorial Hospital to the Medical Director, 29 October 1942.
159 The Bulawayo Bantu Community Association was one of the various African associations that were mainly concerned with African welfare in African townships. Led by African middle-class professionals such as teachers, pastors, police offices and businessmen, such organisations had the approval of the government and in most cases the government gave them a sympathetic ear.
160 NAZ ZBP 2/1/3, The Bulawayo Bantu Community Association, memorandum to the National Health Services Commission, no date.
161 NAZ LG 12/7/29, Resident Location Nurses. Entry into their quarters, 6 October 1944–18 March 1946.
162 NAZ ZBP 2/1/1, National Health Services Commission, Letter from the Coloured Services League, 13 August 1945.
163 P. R. Warhurst, 'The history of race relations in Rhodesia', *Zambezia*, 3: 1 (1973), pp. 15–19.
164 Warhurst, 'The history of race relations in Rhodesia', pp. 15–19.
165 On how hospital spaces blurred the boundaries between races in Rhodesia see C. Masakure, 'Government hospitals as a microcosm: Integration and segregation in Salisbury Hospital, Rhodesia, 1890s–1950', in J. L. Stevens Crawshaw, I. Benyovsky Latin and K. Vongsathorn (eds), *Tracing hospital boundaries: Integration and segregation in southeastern Europe and beyond, 1050–1970* (Leiden: Brill, 2020), pp. 246–69.
166 NAZ S 1173/170, Salisbury Hospital, 1924–1936, letter from the Secretary of Salisbury Hospital to the Medical Director, 29 November 1928.
167 See H. Sweet and A. Digby, 'Race, identity and nursing profession in South Africa, c.1850–1958', in B. Mortimer and S. McGann (eds), *New direction in nursing history: International perspectives* (New York: Routledge, 2005), pp. 109–24; Burns, 'A man is a clumsy thing who does not know how to handle a sick person', pp. 695–717 and Marks, *Divided sisterhood*.

168 See A. Stoler and F. Cooper, 'Between metropole and colony: Rethinking a research agenda', in A. Stoler and F. Cooper (eds), *Tensions of empire: Colonial cultures in a bourgeois world* (Berkeley: University of California Press, 1997), pp. 1–56.
169 Warhurst, 'The history of race relations in Rhodesia', pp. 15–19.
170 For more see J. McCulloch, *Black peril, white virtue: Sexual crime in Southern Rhodesia* (Indiana University Press: Bloomington, 2000), J. Pape, 'Black and white: The "perils of sex" in colonial Zimbabwe', *Journal of Southern African Studies*, 16: 4 (1990), pp. 699–720 and N. Etherington, 'Natal's black rape cases of the 1870s', *Journal of Southern African Studies*, 15: 1 (1988), pp. 36–53.
171 See McCulloch, *Black peril, white virtue*.
172 See Marks, *Divided sisterhood*.
173 Sweet and Digby, 'Race, identity and the nursing profession in South Africa', p. 111.
174 Captain W. A. Whittington, Southern Rhodesia Legislative Assembly Debates, volume 24, 1944, p. 871.
175 Burns, 'A man is a clumsy thing who does not know how to handle a sick person', pp. 695–717.
176 B. J. Mnyanda, *In search of truth: A commentary on certain aspects of Southern Rhodesian Native policy* (Bombay: Hind Kitabs, 1954), p. 41.
177 See Marks, 'We were men nursing men', pp. 177–204; Burns, 'A man is a clumsy thing who does not know how to handle a sick person', pp. 695–717; and L. A. Jackson, *Surfacing up: Psychiatry and social order in colonial Zimbabwe, 1908–1968* (Ithaca, NY: Cornell University Press, 2005).
178 It must be noted that the training of male qualified nurses was only instituted in 1966, both in European and in African training schools.
179 For more see Masakure, 'One of the most serious problems'.
180 For more on this see Schmidt, *Peasants, traders, and wives*.
181 Marks, 'We were men nursing men', pp. 177–204.
182 For South Africa, see for example, Burns, 'A man is a clumsy thing who does not know how to handle a sick person', pp. 695–717.
183 NAZ ZBP 2/1/3, National Health Services Commission, Memorandum by C. S. Mitchell, Salisbury Hospital Secretary to the National Health Services Commission, 25 October 1945.
184 NAZ ZBP 2/1/3, National Health Services Commission, Plof. W. Nirdjesjo, Mnene Mission to the National Health Services Commission, 7 December 1945.
185 *The African Parade*, January 1959.
186 *The African Parade*, August 1958.

3

'Our kitchen days are over ... We can no longer continue the tradition of our predecessors': Taking up nursing as a career option, c. 1950 to the 1960s

In the wake of the social and economic transformations occurring in Southern Rhodesia in the post-Second World War period,[1] government officials started to adjust nursing services in the colony by availing the State Registered Nursing (SRN) qualification to non-Europeans. This was done in two ways. First, the government began offering bursaries to young African women to train at McCord Hospital in South Africa.[2] Second, the government initiated training non-Europeans as SRNs in Rhodesia. As a result, the first cohort of coloured student nurses commenced training at Princess Margaret Hospital in 1953.[3] The cohort of coloured nurses qualified on 3 September 1957.[4] In 1959, *The Central African Journal of Medicine* carried a story about the first coloured nurse who qualified at Princess Margaret Hospital to join Government Nursing Services. Helen Barbara Rhoades was not just one of the first cohort to train at Princess Margaret Hospital in 1953, but also proceeded to Britain where she gained a Midwifery Certificate.[5] Furthermore, African nursing students began training as SRNs at Harari and Impilo hospitals five years later in 1958.[6] The nursing programme for Africans began with fifteen students – three from Northern Rhodesia, one from Nyasaland and the rest from Southern Rhodesia.[7] Forty-five students were admitted each year and Gelfand clearly states that in 1979, Harari Hospital (Gomo), together with the nurses trained there, had 'saved countless lives, given relief for many and cured an untold number of men, women and children'.[8]

Yet casting state policy as the most significant factor in making it easier for women to enter the nursing profession in the 1950s obscures more than it reveals. It masks African agency, especially the failure to appreciate the disparate yet interrelated motives behind nurses selecting nursing as a career option. Thus, I argue that as much as the government preferred female nurses, a history of African nurses in Rhodesia must consider a systematic analysis of motives for choosing nursing.

Using oral accounts from nurses as the main evidentiary base, I examine the various reasons for embracing nursing as a preferred career option. Amongst other things, I consider the link between the motive to join the nursing profession and the various identities that were constituted by African female nurses during the time under discussion. Horwitz argues that an examination of women's motives for choosing nursing as a profession revealed how nurses defined themselves as well as the significance of the process in shaping their nursing professional identity.[9] Notably, I consider professional identity as being more than knowing the art of taking care of the infirm, it encompasses *inter alia*, having the prestige that comes with the knowledge of nursing science. Professional identity also includes the authority associated with being a nurse in the post-Second World War era. All these were not new as they were a continuation of the prestige and authority that came to be associated with hospital work from the beginning of the introduction of colonial hospitals. However, the time under study witnessed the construction of hospitals and clinics, increases in the number of trainees, and the opening up of SRN training to non-Europeans, which made nurses more visible within African communities. As a result, a close analysis of the women's narratives shifts the angle of analysis from colonial historical stereotypes defining these African women as mere purveyors of colonial ideas to one that appreciates the agency evident in the nurses' shaping of what it meant to be a nurse in Rhodesia. Hence, just as with the earlier generations of hospital workers, this identity – *kuva mukoti* (being a nurse) – enabled them to differentiate themselves from vernacular nursing practitioners, and from other working colonial women such as teachers, typists, nannies and factory workers.

The privileging of women's motives for choosing nursing as a preferred career option, even though opportunities were limited, opens up a new analytical paradigm in the analysis of the social and economic changes taking place amongst Rhodesian African women during the post-1950 period. The time under study witnessed the opening up of socio-economic opportunities, facilitated by the nursing profession, which had been severely limited for earlier generations. One was expected to have passed the Standard VI level to study and be a nurse during the time under discussion, a condition which resulted in few women acquiring the qualifications to enter nursing. The limited entrance of African women into nursing also resulted from the Rhodesian government's policy of restricting education for Africans. Nonetheless, the few women who qualified to enter nursing schools and ended up working in hospitals were able to constitute a sense of their competency and make considerable contributions to society. Furthermore, social mobility was also closely related to this transformation. Traditionally, various African women would enter into what historian Michael West termed the 'African middle class' through their association with male suitors, parents or other relatives.[10] However, professions such as nursing and teaching gave women another option for social mobility. Nursing enabled African women to move up the social ladder, which is a development that seemed distant for most African women before the Second World War.[11]

Focusing on women's hopes and aspirations also gives us an opportunity to examine the rate at which assumptions about women's roles and work were changing in Rhodesia from the 1950s onwards. Nurse Christine Mawema captured the potential offered by nursing and its role in extending the professionalisation of women in Rhodesia, as noted in her statement made in an interview with *The African Parade* in 1960 that: 'Our kitchen days are over … We can no longer continue the tradition of our predecessors. We just want to be treated as equals with our men and we will do it, I tell you!'[12] Christine Mawema, the wife of Michael Mawema, one of the early nationalists in African politics, spoke in 1960 at a time when African nationalists were beginning to push for independence, thus showing how she also perceived the African anticolonial activism in search for better and humane treatment as part of women's struggle. Christine Mawema, who at times attended political rallies alongside her husband,[13] suggested in her views that differences were emerging between the older generation of women and the younger ones. Thus, on one hand, the generation of the 1950s and 1960s, as represented by Mawema, viewed their grandmothers and mothers as defined by their confinement to the kitchen and the domestic space. On the other hand, the *dare* (men's court) is a male space, with any man who spent most of his time in the kitchen being derided as *chinzvengamutsvairo* (the broom dodger). This idea that the kitchen was the woman's space was further buttressed by missionary education and its resultant moulding of African family life along western Victorian standards.[14] However, from the 1950s onwards, formal employment presented new opportunities that allowed women to push the boundaries of what was expected of them. Mawema and her generation of professional women hoped and aspired that their new-found status would enable them to be treated on an equal basis with men. Therefore, I argue that the professionalisation of African women as SRNs in Rhodesia gives us a platform from which to examine the ways that African women's everyday lives were being redefined from the traditional domestic responsibilities and by their association with men, either as suitors, husbands or as their male relatives. Public spaces, such as hospitals, became new sites that enabled African women to reshape and negotiate their relations and move up the social ladder in post-Second World War Rhodesia.

Imagining the possibilities offered by the nursing profession

It is important to contextualise the social environment that made it possible for African women to imagine and experience the possibilities offered by nursing. This is significant since, in Rhodesia as in South Africa, the extension of trained nursing to African women was influenced by the prevailing gender norms in both white and African societies.[15] The tasks and skills that young women performed and learned within their households were transferable to hospital settings and the nursing profession. Traditionally, young women helped with everyday household chores within African societies. What is most important for this study is that elderly women worked with young women in taking care of and nursing the infirm.[16] Nurses such as Wendy Mwamuka underscored the significance of the Shona tradition in imparting the desire within women to enter the profession. Wendy Mwamuka's specific experience with her grandmother, who was the village midwife, played a role in her choosing to work in hospitals as noted in her statement:

> I started as a midwife in 1952 at Bonda Mission Hospital. By that time, I had finished Standard Six at Bonda Mission School. It was not a difficult choice for me at all because my grandmother who was a *nyamukuta* (traditional midwife) started teaching me birthing practices at the age of 16. It seems it was part of our family tradition as she had learnt from her mother. She began by showing me traditional medicines. On some occasions, I would tag along when she was called to deliver babies … That is where my interests in midwifery and later on nursing came from. This was my first school and it made it easier for me to adjust to clinical midwifery. By the time I started working as a midwife at the Mission Hospital, I was well knowledgeable with birthing practices.[17]

Wendy Mwamuka's case was an exception as many lacked experience in traditional midwifery practices. Still, they emphasised the traditional division of labour as a significant component of their initial training. Thus, nursing in Rhodesia was a woman's space, where women had more control over their work as compared to other professions such as teaching. Furthermore, there was less interest amongst young men to enter nursing. As Kufa Mutoro, with over 40 years' experience working as a nursing orderly, explained: 'Many young men thought that nursing was for women and very few were ambitious to work in hospitals. Many preferred working in what were considered male professions, especially in industry. My job as a nursing orderly was to do the heavy work that women could not do. Nursing was mainly a woman's sphere.'[18] The gendering of the profession gave women an advantage over men who might have considered the possibility of working in hospitals. In addition, the fact that young women who took up nursing were in their mid-teens and had been initiated into the art and culture of caring for the infirm indicates the ingrained gender roles already existing in the society.[19] Undeniably, the domestic chores women performed instilled a sense of confidence that they could achieve similar tasks as nurses. This then constituted the imagined future, which coincided with the sharp increase in the need for African nurses in Rhodesia during the post-Second World War period.

Households, mission stations, schools and hospitals also played a prominent role in preparing young women for nursing. Missionary education reinforced the idea that African women were most suitable for taking up nursing. Mission schools played a significant role in the lives of many Africans, with the interviewed nurses underscoring the critical way in which missionaries nurtured ideas about taking up the profession. In addition, it was at mission hospitals and clinics where some of the nurses commenced the entrance into the profession as nursing assistants.

Acquiring education – *kufunda* – was not an easy task for African women. Not only did African parents prefer educating boys at the expense of girls, but the system was also heavily rigged against Africans.[20] In Rhodesia there was a systematic privileging of white students with regards to educational opportunities and resource allocation. West argued that although the post-Second World War era saw the reassessment of policy on African education, there was still a considerable bottleneck in African education that resulted in only a minority of Africans managing to complete their education.[21] Statistics from the 1960s and 1970s provide us with a clear picture of the limited educational opportunities available to Africans. John Pape noted that during the early 1960s, less than 2 per cent of all African students completed nine years in school and less than 0.5 per cent completed eleven years. By 1977, for every 1,000 African children in Rhodesia, 250 never went to school. Of the remaining 750 only 337 completed primary school. Of these 337 about sixty entered secondary school, and of those sixty only three finished their 'A' (Advanced) level.[22] These figures represented all Africans and, worse still, the probability of young African women being in the remaining 750 was lower. Only a few young women managed to complete eleven years in school.[23] The colonial administration limited the availability of education to a few Africans and in the process affected the prospects of social mobility for the majority of the African population. Thus, for those who had the chance to acquire western education, *kufunda* was a once in a lifetime opportunity not to be missed.

The significance of mission schools in moulding imaginings about nursing should not be underestimated. The mission school curriculum for African girls consisted of home economics, hygiene, baby care and at times obstetrics. In addition, missionaries structured their education in such a way that it prepared them for teaching or nursing. Here, the Wayfarer Movement immediately comes to mind.[24] Youth movements, as social engineering projects, inculcated *chirungu/chingezi* (westernisation) amongst young Africans.[25] Missionaries dismantled African cultures by using youth movements as platforms to offer African youth an alternative to initiation schools.[26] Elizabeth Schmidt noted that the Wayfarer Movement in Rhodesia was concerned with the development of moral and upstanding young women and offering appropriate training for their future role as elite Christian wives and mothers. Premised on the belief that 'idle hands and minds were fertile grounds for the devil's temptations',[27] the Wayfarer Movement promoted activities that would occupy girls' leisure time productively and taught them ways in which Christian ideas could be worked out in daily life.[28] While missionaries thought they were just training them to be good Christian wives, some young women, such as Stella Munemo, conceptualised the Wayfarer Movement differently. They perceived it as a stepping stone to opportunities that were otherwise closed to most rural young women. Stella Munemo noted that her assistant role to the head nurse as a young Wayfarer, made her realise what she wanted to do with her life after completing school. She commented that:

> I was a leader in our group. One day the head nurse at the mission clinic came to us and asked me whether I was interested in helping her in the clinic on Saturday mornings. I said yes without hesitation, and that is how I got involved with the work at the clinic. She was very instrumental in my application to Harari Hospital nursing school, as she wanted someone more qualified to help her. I never returned as I got married a few months after finishing school. I feel that if it was not for Wayfarer and the opportunity it gave me to realise my potential, I would have languished in the village.[29]

Thus, women such as Stella Munemo used the experiences from the Wayfarer Movement and their connections within the movement to position themselves towards accessing the limited opportunities available to young African women. Stella Munemo was not surprised that a significant number of girls within her cohort went into either nursing or teaching. Hence, an array of experiences such as the involvement in colonial and mission education-based youth movements and subjection to a gendered curriculum were important in making it easier for African women to adjust to nursing.

Becoming a nurse and the forging of the nursing identity

There were other factors which motivated African women to choose the nursing profession. Role models and the prestige associated with nursing figured prominently in nurses' recollections. Nurses drew inspiration from an earlier generation of mission-trained nursing orderlies and nursing assistants who had opened the path for them in the pre-Second World War era.[30] These trailblazers had shown the determination and will to succeed, a condition that the later generations wished to emulate. Christina Banda is emblematic of such women. Born on 16 January 1935, she did her nurse training in Livingstone, Northern Rhodesia, between 1955 and 1958. She came back to Bulawayo in 1958 and worked at a number of hospitals in rural and urban areas. In recalling the reasons why she chose nursing as a preferred profession, Christina Banda noted that her teenage days were marked by an admiration of the manner in which nurses practised their craft and conducted themselves. Hence, her determination to be a nurse:

> As we were growing up, we used to admire nursing orderlies, how they conducted their work. Bandaging wounds, taking temperatures and giving shots. That is one of the many things that I admired about nurses. By the time I went for my secondary education, I had made up my mind that I wanted to be a nurse.[31]

Christina Banda's remarks point to one of the crucial distinctions between nurses and other professional women: their work. Having access to western knowledge and especially western knowledge centring on disease diagnosis, healing and taking care of the infirm, elevated them above other professions such as teaching and administration clerks. Thus, witnessing the success status of those already in the profession and having access to hospital technologies and the skill to use such technologies, made nursing attractive to the young African women.

Nursing orderlies and nursing assistants were not just ordinary people within their communities. They were examples of the possibilities offered by formal employment in a racist and oppressive society. Nursing orderlies and nursing assistants were perceived by most Africans as an embodiment of what Africans could achieve if given the opportunity. Various young women who grew up in the post-Second World War period considered nursing orderlies and assistants, and the world they represented, as a source of inspiration. Nomsa Makoni, just as all of my informants, admired the early generation of hospital workers who, like her aunt and her cohort, worked at the mission hospital in her area. According to Nomsa Makoni, her aunt 'motivated young girls in our village to think about working at the clinic, and there were a number of us who admired her work'.[32] Apart from admiring and hoping to emulate her aunt's work, Nomsa Makoni was fascinated by the white dresses that the nursing assistants wore. She explained that her aunt projected an image of cleanliness, neatness and someone in command of her life:

> I was not only attracted by her work, but also by her attire – the white dress she used to wear. We used to see nurses elegantly dressed and with their makeup. I said I want to be like them, be smartly dressed, have access to expensive oils and perfume, my hair nicely done and I will look glamorous and beautiful. Every day I saw her in the nursing uniform I envied her and I imagined myself becoming a nurse one day.[33]

Tsitsi Chinamasa also suggested similar reasons for having been attracted to nursing, 'I thought of becoming a nurse especially because of the conduct of nurses in public and the way they used to dress. They always looked clean in white dresses, and it gave a good impression to the patients that they must always be clean.'[34] Bodily cleanliness, both in appearance and in dress, was very intriguing and important in the narratives of nurses. Hence, African nurses in Rhodesia, just as African nurses in South Africa, viewed the white uniform as a symbol of higher status and prestige.[35]

The centrality of nurses' conduct and appearance in oral narratives can be linked to the construction of the nursing identity. The nursing identity was closely linked with the circulating ideas of hygiene. Indeed, nurses led by example as preachers of the gospel of cleanliness and their homes were expected to be clean. Cleanliness and hygiene were embedded in the discourses on Africans' cleanliness. Scholars have shown how cleanliness was used as a marker of difference between colonials and their subjects.[36] Missionaries and colonial officials considered it their duty to 'civilise' Africans through the gospel of cleanliness. As argued by Timothy Burke, the notions of cleanliness, appearance and bodily behaviour became increasingly powerful within colonised African communities in the 1930s. According to Burke, the growing power of these new behaviours among emerging African elites and whites can be explained as signs of struggle between 'tradition and modern life, African and European ways, heathenism and Christianity'.[37] This pedagogy of cleanliness and manners had entrenched itself as a standard component of African education by the 1940s and had a tremendous effect on conventions of self-representation in Rhodesia.[38] These notions became part of everyday life as more Africans gained greater access to material goods. Hence, the cleanliness and hygienic nature of nurses expressed through the mode of dress was paradoxically an implicit reaction to the racist stereotype of the African body as a diseased and dirty one, and an appropriation that nurses used to counter the stereotypes projected by colonials.[39]

Nurses deployed similar ideas on cleanliness, which functioned as a marker of difference between professional women and the 'other' non-formally employed women. The white uniforms, brown stockings and brown shoes that the nurses wore made a significant statement regarding access to new forms of status and the constitution of one's identity. A key point that features prominently in the nurses' narratives focused on the respect commanded by the uniforms and how these uniforms stood out as symbols of class and status amongst African women. Nurses were thus respected in their communities because of the dignity – *chiremera* – associated with both the nursing uniform and profession. Again, Nomsa Makoni recalled that: 'We were always clean, spotlessly clean.'[40] Furthermore, Nelia Ncube, who trained in the early 1970s at Impilo Hospital in Bulawayo, stated that nurses had such a high status in the past to the extent that when someone driving their car saw a nurse walking home in the rain, they would stop and offer the nurse a ride. This was because 'the white uniform was held in higher esteem than what is happening today. When going to or coming from work, people would say, yes! Those are nurses. They are there to serve the community.'[41] Estha Mawoyo echoed similar sentiments in her statement that, 'Most of us became nurses because of the reverence that came with the uniform and the nature of our profession. The uniform gave us respect and everywhere, from rural areas to urban areas, African nurses were well respected during those days.'[42] The significance of the uniform is also reflected in Estha Mawoyo's answer to my question on whether there would have been any difference if nurses practised their craft in civilian clothing; she was adamant that it would have been difficult to identify who was or was not a nurse if they were not wearing their uniforms. Wearing uniforms, having badges and brooches that signalled one's nursing rank, as well as having a Nurse Watch pinned to the uniform, were affirmations of the nurses' right to undertake certain tasks within hospitals. As J. Craick noted, 'the uniform of each occupation conveys an immediately perceived sense of skills and knowledge as well as expectations of the relationship between the worker and others'.[43] Hence, nurses' uniforms allowed patients, colleagues and their communities to easily identify the nurses and, by implication, to recognise their skills and knowledge.

Uniforms, as specialised types of clothing for dressing, are used to announce a particular set of identities.[44] The African nurses' wearing of a particular type of uniform that was also a universal one provided an opportunity to identify with the global image of nurses. The work and uniforms meant that the African nurses were part of a sisterhood. The nurses affirmed their entry into the global sisterhood through wearing white uniforms just as their European and coloured counterparts. This idea, however, should be balanced with everyday work experiences. Nurses, as Shula Marks aptly demonstrated, were part of a divided sisterhood that was experienced both structurally and racially.[45] Race played a significant factor in determining one's position within hospitals in Rhodesia, just as in South Africa. The hospital structure was organised in such a way that nurses of European origin were more privileged, followed by nurses of Asian origin and coloured nurses, with African nurses at the base of this hierarchy. In this case, therefore, the differences between nurses, even though they belonged to a global sisterhood, made this shared experience elusive. In addition, rather than enhance their position, uniforms ironically made it easier for their seniors, doctors and hospital administrators to boss African nurses around. The following statement made by Estha Mawoyo is instructive:

> Nursing students were easily identifiable by the absence of badges on their epaulette and it made them more vulnerable to be used in house duties

than other nurses with badges. Even if you have badges, you might find that junior doctors just look at you, as if one does not know what she is doing.[46]

Nevertheless, the environment here reflected a military hierarchy, which meant that the absence of badges on the African nurses' epaulettes indicated the nurses' junior status. This ultimately indicated that, while uniforms, just as in South Africa, meant the nurses were part of the nursing sisterhood, the ascribed junior status meant that African nurses were part of a divided sisterhood.[47]

Some of the nurses' responses reflected their struggles in defining their professional identity and distinguishing nurses from other professionals such as teachers. The responses also distinguished older nurses from the younger generation of nurses. In this way, nurses also underscored one of the factors that drew them into nursing as the philanthropic nature of the profession. Some argued that healing the sick and helping the infirm formed part of their religious responsibility.[48] Jane Mushando, born in 1941 at Mt Selinda Hospital, a key health centre in the South East of the country, run by the American Board Mission, explained the reasons why she and her friends went for nurse training in this way:

> It was natural for me that I would go into nursing. I never had any doubts with it ... As a mother, I love seeing babies being born but most importantly, I felt it was my religious responsibility to help the sick, especially those without relatives to take care of them. That is why I decided to go into nursing.[49]

Jane Mushando reiterated further that she had no regrets in taking up nursing, as that was what she always wanted to do, and that if given another chance, she would take up nursing again. This is noted in Jane Mushando's statement that, 'Yes, I will still take up nursing because I love the job. You know, since I retired, I have always been on locum, being called here and there to help with the staffing situation at the hospital. At times, I would say that I do not want to do this anymore, but because I love the job, I have always been coming back to it, as locum, a fall back.'[50]

Laiza Shumba, a contemporary of Jane Mushando, had a similar story. She stated that taking care of the infirm and healing the sick was one of her wishes, and emphasised that nursing was a calling.[51] Her response to my question on whether there were other options that were available for African women, clearly revealed the opportunities, the nature of the conditions that existed during that time, and the reasons for choosing nursing as a profession, as noted here:

> Teaching of course. This was one of the options available to us as young girls. You see, during our days there were very few jobs available for us women. It is either you have to go into teaching or nursing and clerical work. However, clerical work became open a bit late for us Africans. When it came to teaching, I just did not like the idea of spending the whole day with children. You would spend the whole day talking and talking. There is nothing wrong about being with children but I preferred being with patients at the hospital. Maybe it was the idea that you can immediately see how you are investing your time. Patients getting well and you feel good about your contribution. Of course, as with working in hospital, people die and sometimes you get sad. Nevertheless, it is always a bundle of joy either delivering a new baby or seeing somebody recovering. With schoolchildren, you just have to be patient; you get to know the results of your work way later in life. There is nothing wrong with teaching but I preferred being with the patients in hospital. Healing the sick was more satisfactory for me.[52]

Therefore, Laiza Shumba and Jane Mushando, who represented an early generation of trained nurses, viewed nursing as a marker of difference with other professional women. In addition, nursing differentiated them from the other women who worked in the colonial industries and on farms.

There is no doubt that the younger generations of nurses had more professional opportunities open to them than the earlier generations. The 1970s presented African women with more choices of professions and these included journalism, accounting and secretarial work. Nevertheless, younger nurses highlighted the philanthropic nature of the profession as one of the motivating factors for choosing it. Maidei Madziwa, who entered the profession in 1973, underlined altruism as the factor that convinced her to take up nursing. She also emphasised the joy that she felt in doing her work, the centrality of nursing to her life, and how she desired to contribute towards healing the infirm:

> I have always been interested in this profession. I think my main attraction to nursing was that I wanted to help healing people. I really feel that there are people out there who put everything on the wire for the sake of the sick. It is my calling, something I feel I was born to do and I will never regret being a nurse. I just love the profession, being able to see patients getting well. At least I feel that I am contributing something to my community.[53]

Being a nurse was life fulfilling for Maidei Madziwa and she belonged to the same sisterhood as the earlier generation of nurses. Estha Mawoyo, who, at the time of the interviews was in her late forties, also raised similar compassionate sentiments in her statement that, 'Nursing is an honourable profession, and the greatest encouragement one can get is from the patient and knowing that one's care and attention has helped to bring healthy and happy results.'[54] She stressed the need to be passionate about the work and be prepared to work for long hours and night duties.

The older nurses differentiated themselves from later generations of nurses through highlighting their dedication to nursing and the philanthropic nature of the profession. They argued that, unlike younger nurses, they were eager to serve their communities. These nurses, who were probably frustrated with the changes that took place in the country's economy and the health sector's hospital system in the 1990s, which were being felt during the time of the research,[55] and owing to their recollection of years as younger women, insinuated that they were prepared to work overtime and under harsh conditions as well as with limited resources when compared with most junior nurses. These senior nurses projected themselves as 'true nurses'.[56] However, the junior nurses argued that they were equally dedicated to the profession and their presence within clinical spaces did not undermine the traditional nursing identity, for they viewed nursing as an instrument to serve their communities just as their senior compatriots. Tsitsi Chinamasa underlined younger nurses' commitment to the profession and their continued intention to serve the community through taking care of the infirm:

> There are a lot problems and frustrations being experienced in the profession. Thus, many of our seniors quickly point fingers at junior nurses. Young women have so many options open to them but the fact that they chose nursing is an indicator of their commitment to the profession.[57]

There is no doubt that the crisis experienced within the health sector from the 1990s influenced the responses that were provided by the nurses. In addition, it is my conviction that generational differences affected the informants' responses as it was mainly older and senior nurses who maintained that they were more passionate about their job than junior and younger nurses. Older nurses constructed junior nurses as apathetic and insincere to their cause. The underlying argument by older nurses is that nursing has changed, 'it is no longer what it used to be'.[58] Such arguments are part of daily contestations over the professional identity of nursing.

The quest for respectability and middle-class status

As early as 1944, three African nursing assistants showed the possibilities that could be gained from their social position within colonial society. The nursing assistants, working at the then Location Clinic in Harari Township, nearly filed a lawsuit against the Location Superintendent. The lawsuit, which was prevented from pursuing its full course, was an unprecedented move carried out by African women against the local authority. The act showed a sign of self-confidence by African women in a racially oppressive colonial society.[59] At the same time, the case offers us an opportunity to appreciate some of the ways in which elite African women overtly challenged colonial authority.[60] In fact, the case illustrates the lengths African women were willing to go in negotiating their position in Rhodesia. These women's social standing within the community as nurses enabled them to question colonial policies and assert their right to association and freedom of movement. Such an incident also reveals that educated African women were fully conscious of their status within African communities and prepared to use the legal route in an attempt to make sure that they were duly respected.

The story unfolded in this way. At about five o'clock in the morning on Monday, 25 September 1944, two African municipal police raided the house occupied by three African nursing assistants searching for members of the Royal Air Force (RAF).[61] The colonial society limited racial mixing and as such, many white Rhodesians loathed the thought that some European men were having relationships with African women. African men also felt that it was improper for African women to have relationships with white men. However, the crux of the matter was that members of the RAF were not permitted to overstay in the Location under the Salisbury City bylaws.[62] A part of the testimony from one of the police officers read:

I first knocked at the door and someone said who are you? I replied I am police officer of the Location. A person then came to door and unlocked it. I noticed it was one of the nurses. She asked me what I was looking for. I said I was looking for a RAF soldier who used to frequent these premises. The nurse walked backward and said come in. I followed her into the dining room and looked through the open door into the bedroom, which she had just left. I saw no one. The nurse then knocked on the door of the other bedroom and spoke to other nurses in a language I do not understand. The nurse came out of her room and I looked through the open door but saw none therein. Thereafter, I walked out of the cottage followed by both nurses who remained on the veranda talking in their own language. They did not protest at any time against my entering the premises. It was quite light when I made the search and it was unnecessary to have an artificial light to carry out my search. I left the premises with the other police boy (man) and went to report to the sergeant.[63]

The police officer maintained that there was no malice or jealousy on his part for conducting the search. In addition, he swore that he did not tell anyone. He had only reported the case to the Superintendent and had no clue as to how the information had spread throughout the Location. Feeling aggrieved and humiliated by the invasion of privacy, the nurses complained to the Superintendent of the Location. In an effort to assert their difference to other women in the Location, the nursing orderlies insisted on seeing him in private. The Superintendent, however, turned down their request and maintained that they had to follow the procedure as required of other Africans and report their grievances in the presence of Europeans and Africans alike.[64]

Even though the police officer did not find the European airmen, there is the probability that nursing orderlies frequently disregarded Location rules.[65] During that weekend an airman had been spotted with one of the nurses at a dance in the afternoon, and the nurses, in their statements, did not refute that the airmen had stayed in the Location for more than twelve hours.[66] Despite the fact that they might have broken the rule, the nursing assistants emphasised their right to privacy and the need to be treated with respect. Part of the letter from their lawyer read:

> The natives (nurse assistants) complain that they have been disgraced in their character, status and feeling as a result of what has occurred, and that they object most strongly to the fact of the raid and the manner in which it

was carried out and they object further most strongly to the conduct of the Location Superintendent after the raid.[67]

The nurses, who felt that they had been disrespected and labelled immoral, instructed their lawyers to demand a proper apology from the Superintendent. The apology had to contain an admission that the allegations made against the nurses were absolutely and entirely unfounded.

While the nursing assistants were unsuccessful in their quest, the threat of a lawsuit can be used as a window into analysing 'elite' women's perceptions of the self. The nurses invoked the human rights discourse, the need to be treated with dignity and their right to privacy.[68] Furthermore, the effort was a direct challenge to the Superintendent's authority and power to authorise the raid. The letter continued thus:

> They (nursing assistants) require to know under what authority the superintendent made the raid, and what powers he, or the location police had to make the raid under these circumstances. They state that the least that could have occurred was that they should have been questioned about the matter, particularly since as nurses their social status is considerable in the Location.[69]

The nursing assistants, who perceived themselves as part of the privileged elites, demanded the right to be treated with respect and dignity. They were, however, not the first women to be treated like this in the Location, neither were they the last.[70] What is interesting to note is that the nursing assistants argued for individual rights as prominent women in the Location. There is no evidence that they also advocated rights of other women who resided in the Location.

Although the above case was an exception, significant to appreciate is that nurses who entered the profession from the 1950s onwards had similar confidence in their capabilities and of the possibilities that came with formal employment. Fictional writings and oral sources depict nursing narratives that linked the profession with the 'advancement' of African women. Though highly contested, nurses linked this 'advancement' with the quest for respectability and improved social status. Nursing provided stability, brought respect and enabled women to be in charge of their lives. The nurses argued that, while becoming a nurse was a personal 'advancement', the progress was representative of the 'advancement' of African women in general. Yvonne Vera, in her fictional account of Bulawayo portrayed in *Butterfly Burning* (1998), illuminated the meaning of nursing to many young women during the 1950s. Nursing symbolised something new and liberating as depicted in Yvonne Vera's outline of the story of the character, Phephelapi, a woman in her mid-twenties who had the chance to go to the nursing school at United School Hospital, Bulawayo. She grew up in the poor neighbourhood of Makokoba and yearned for something new and life changing. Vera suggested that for Phephelapi, 'it is not being a nurse which matters, but the movement forward – the embrace into something new and untried ... She is going to be the first to train if the occasion allows her.'[71] Undoubtedly, many changes were taking place in the 1940s and 1950s. Educational opportunities, though limited, were fast expanding, enabling Phephelapi and her generation to look forward to the future with an anticipation that their socio-economic conditions would change for the better.

The nursing profession provided a new avenue for African women in an environment that limited their opportunities on the basis of race and gender. The 1950s and 1960s generation of young women felt the same way. Nursing was prestigious and represented progress as Phaina Nyanhanda said:

> During those days going to a nursing school was something so special. With limited opportunities available to Africans, you would have moved up by being a nurse. I remember when I entered nursing school, it was an affirmation that girls can also earn a salary and contribute to the wellbeing of the family.[72]

By the middle of the twentieth century, African women were beginning to break new ground and show that they were on equal terms with men. Teresa Barnes noted the changes that took place in the industrial sector where the post-Second World War period's industrial expansion compelled employers to ditch labour bottlenecks that had existed for a long time and accept 'native females' as new employees.[73] African women's presence also began to be felt within professional employment. Phaina Nyanhanda and her generation demonstrated that they could move up the social ladder on their own. There was a feeling, within the Rhodesian African communities of the 1950s, of progress and that if given an opportunity, Africans could achieve the same as Europeans. In 1954, a letter to *The African Parade*, one of the most influential African magazines, pointed out that:

> Admittedly, the effect of urbanisation on some has been detrimental. On others, it has been otherwise. While there is the loafer, the spiv, the criminal with a perverted mind, you have at the same time the enterprising individual who cannot only hold his own in any sphere where opportunities exist but is both in character and enterprise a national asset. For instance, while the emancipation of women has produced the 'skokian queen' and the prostitute, it has also created the woman who is conscious of her dignity, her right in the community and her duties. Take the countless African women who are earning their living by respectable means such as domestic house cleaners, the girls who work in the factories and *the hospital nurses whose services are every whit the bulwark of African progress* [emphasis is mine].[74]

While African elites and members of the middle class were beginning to question racial exclusivity and colonial structures that limited their opportunities through political mobilisations,[75] they were also very critical of their own people whom they argued were dragging Africans down. Such arguments were influenced by Victorian ideals. It is nonetheless important to appreciate how bourgeois domestic ideas were not simply imported concepts that were imposed on Africans by a culturally alien church and politically repressive state. Instead, as Michael West argued, Africans in Rhodesia were active agents in the acculturation process, with both female and male members of the emerging elites voluntarily accepting the ideology of domesticity. Accordingly, African women, whether independently or in conjunction with African men or whites, formed various associations, clubs and societies to facilitate their efforts to become good wives and mothers along the lines of the Victorian model they had internalised. These self-enabling agencies were even more important than the missionary-run and state-supported institutions in forging new concepts of gender roles among elite Africans.[76] As a result, African elites and members of the middle class felt that criminals, '*skokian* queens' (*shebeen* queens)[77] and prostitutes were the bane of African progress. They also perceived the '*skokian* queens' and prostitutes as retrogressive and undermining the Africans' attempt to achieve the same status as Europeans. Nonetheless, professionals such as nurses were considered a national asset. The nationalist, Edison Sithole, captured this feeling of African progress in general and women's advancement in a speech he made in 1958:

> If one looks today into the teaching and nursing fields one would be amazed to see the vast changes that have taken place amongst the African folk women of Southern Rhodesia … The number of women qualifying as nurses, teachers etc., brings home the fact that women are not inferior to men. I looked through final examination papers of higher nursing, believe me it is not a question of having trousers or dresses in order to pass it.[78]

Such a statement that praised African women's achievement resonated with the ideals upheld in independent Zimbabwe. African communities appreciated the rare achievement.

A discussion on the prestige associated with nursing should also focus on the role played by financial rewards as an immediate pull factor to the profession. Unlike student teachers, student nurses were paid stipends while training. As a result, young women were earning better salaries than most men within a few months in training.[79] The stipend was higher in comparison to the majority of workers' wages, yet there was a gendered and racial disparity regarding wages within the health sector. This is noted in the reality that there was a disparity between male and female trainee orderlies in spite of both genders being exposed to the same curriculum and expected to perform the same job description, as Table 3.1 shows.

Such salary discrepancies were based on the assumption that men were the breadwinners in households and thus deserved better remuneration than women. In addition to the gendered disparity in salaries, there was also a race-based determination of salaries. Colonial policy ensured that Africans were the least paid irrespective of their educational qualifications, with the coloureds and people of Asian

Table 3.1 Salaries per month: African student orderlies (1958)

Year of study	Male student	Female student
First	£ 8 15s	£ 7 5s
Second	£ 9 5s	£ 7 10s
Third	£ 9 15s	£ 7 17s

Source: F 122/FH/190/55

descent lying in between and receiving a comparatively higher wage than Africans. Table 3.2 shows the wage gaps for trainee nurses in 1958, which were readjusted by a 5 per cent increment for non-Europeans in 1960.

This policy was applied to the trained and full-time nurses. On the one hand, a fully trained and qualified nurse received half the salary of a white temporary nurse or 15 per cent of a permanent white nurse. In addition, it was observed, in 1961 that nurses who were promoted into the Branch 'I' had no chance of reaching the bottom grade of salaries offered to European nurses.[80] On the other hand, coloured nurses earned four-fifths and two-thirds of their white equivalents.[81] Thus, the salaries earned by the African nurses did not match the long and arduous stretches of night duty and laborious work they performed in hospitals. This must have frustrated many African nurses. Nelia Ncube did not hide her indignation with the racialised salary structure at trainee level and as a full time nurse:

> It was unfortunate that we were paid according to the colour of our skin. We were discriminated against and it was so frustrating some time that someone is paid more than you because of their race. We did the same jobs but we got little out of it.[82]

The lower salaries nevertheless placed nurses at a still better off position than the average and marginalised African women. For African nurses, the ability to have full control over their salaries was very significant. It gave them freedom and constituted one of the most important differences between this generation of women and their mothers, who were self-employed. It gave them greater freedom both as daughters and later as wives in the household.

Table 3.2 Salaries: Trainee nurses (1958)

Year of training	African	Coloured	European
First	£ 162	£ 207	£ 264
Second	£ 177	£ 222	£ 282
Third	£ 196	£ 237	£ 300
Fourth	£ 207	£ 252	£ 318

Source: F 122/FH/190/55

Earning salaries reshaped social relations within African nurses' homes. A number of them literally took over family responsibilities such as providing for their families' needs and paying school fees for their siblings.[83] One nurse claimed, 'I bought shoes, clothes and many other things for my family. I paid my brothers' school fees and remained with some money. I made it a point to save a pound a month for the whole year to use to meet urgent family needs.'[84] This employed and salaried status transformed nurses into prestigious, respectable and independent figures in a typical patriarchal society that valued fathers, brothers or husbands in the decision-making process and provision of family needs. This does not imply that there was a breakdown of family structures; rather it reflects an evident reshaping of social relations in which women possessed greater bargaining power within their own families or with lovers and potential suitors. For instance, Phaina Nyanhanda suggested that her ability to bring home a stable salary made her husband treat her in a 'dignified' way. I argue, however, that other nurses might not have had similar experiences as some of my informants suggest.[85] Discrepancies in occupational status, education and, to some extent, values, might have caused tensions in marital relations, especially when the wife's salary was equal to or possibly even higher than that of her husband.

Formal employment also led to the establishment of new forms of relationships with other women. Many of these female nurses were in monogamous relationships and juggled between family life and everyday hospital work, which compelled them to seek help with household chores from their younger siblings or relatives. Others went further than relying on close relatives and employed domestic workers to help manage their households. Phaina Nyanhanda, who drew on her own case and those of her friends, vividly remembered different trends involving helpers and maids. The Shona/Ndebele traditions allowed young girls to stay with their relatives to help with household chores, a tradition that Phaina Nyanhanda suggested was still intact in the 1950s. Nonetheless, Phaina Nyanhanda noticed in the early stages of her marriage that her colleagues preferred employing non-relatives. She pointed out that:

> There is nothing wrong in helping some of your relatives by employing them. However, in most cases you will be courting many problems. Relatives talk too much. They complain about this and that. Heeh, the money is not

enough, heeh I am being used, heeh they do not feed me. They cause so many problems. Therefore, it is better to employ someone who is not your relative. You just agree, this is what I want and this is how much I can afford to give you. If they do not perform as expected, then it is easier to replace them.[86]

The employment of other women was both a status symbol and indicative of a status change for many African women. It epitomised the possibilities that came with formal employment. It also represented the birthing of new sets of relationships between African women in Rhodesia. Undoubtedly, what changed from previous relationships was the mechanism through which some women gained access to other women's labour through a predominantly wage relationship.[87]

A particularly different African nurse and domestic worker employer and employee relationship was also created here. Unlike domestic workers who worked within white households, maids who worked for African nurses virtually became part of the family as they usually shared a bedroom with their employers' children and ate the family food. In most cases, these girls assumed many, if not most of the domestic duties. My informants indicated that they expected their maids to be well versed with domestic chores. Phaina Nyanhanda usually taught her maids 'how to press clothes, cook, and clean properly'.[88] Nevertheless, the fact that a significant number did not employ relatives with the intention of avoiding conflicts, does not mean that relationships between the African nurse employers and their house cleaners were tension free. There were many problems that were encountered by the nurses with many failing to stay with their house cleaners for longer periods. Pregnancies contributed to a high turnover rate, but the primary cause was economic, as interviews revealed that African nurse employers failed to pay attractive wages.[89] The nurses, however, complained that house cleaners used them as stepping-stones to other, better paying jobs.[90] Nonetheless, I argue that by employing and teaching the maids new housekeeping practices, African nurses facilitated the forging of new social and wage-based relationships with fellow African women. At the same time, the fact that the African nurses could afford to employ maids affirmed that they had entered the middle class. Furthermore, a comparison of the Rhodesian conditions with the changes in domestic employment taking place in the post-colonial period is essential in bringing this point home. In his study of domestic work, John Pape argued that the existence of a minority white and an African class with the financial capacity to employ domestic workers was substantially altered in the post-colonial period. The post-colonial era witnessed a broadening of the utilisation of domestic workers as nearly all Zimbabwean black urban households, regardless of their class, became employers of domestic workers.[91] However, the colonial period had been characterised by a tiny minority of the African population, especially professional women, who could afford to employ domestic servants.

Formal employment radically changed women's lives in Rhodesia. An examination of the women's daily consumption patterns and the associated material culture is instructive in outlining how the women took up opportunities presented by paid employment to take charge of their lives. Access to economic resources enabled the African women to set new fashion and consumption trends amongst fellow women in Rhodesia. Nurses were the envy of the town and many young women strived to imitate their fashion trends.[92] Laiza Shumba confirmed this in her recollection of her trainee days:

> I used my money to buy my own supplies, those commodities which my parents could not afford to buy for me. New clothes, wigs, better quality soaps and lotions. Instead of straightening our hair with a hot stone without chemicals, we could now afford to buy hair preparations and shampoos. People will know that this young girl is in charge of her life with the way one presented herself and the way one looked.[93]

Laiza Shumba and her generation perceived the new fashions as symbols of power and respectability. Furthermore, it was liberating for many to be seen and to engage in buying a new dress, a wig, or a new pair of shoes using personal savings and without seeking the approval of the male members of the family.

The manner in which nurses articulated the significance of these new status symbols underlines their achievement of a status change. Most of my informants indicated that cosmetics were part of their conspicuous consumption and that these products made them look beautiful, with the daily access and use enabling them to gain respect within the society.[94] Nevertheless, the use of cosmetics, especially amongst young unmarried nurses, would at times undo what they had tried to achieve. Weinrich's study on Mucheke Township during the 1970s, noted that women with higher social status – nurses, wives of professionals and the wives of railway workers – all used skin lighteners, hair straighteners and cosmetics, including lipstick, while those women who did not have easy access to such cosmetics, criticised cosmetic use amongst the wealthy and labelled them former prostitutes, which suggests that cosmetic use ended up eroding the status of nurses and wives of professionals.[95] It is probable that jealousy and financial problems affecting many families at the time might have played a significant factor in influencing women's responses as presented in Weinrich's study. However, there were also some moral issues associated with cosmetics that date back to the 1930s. There is a long history of the association between heavy cosmetics and low-class women. Burke noted that many 'shebeen queens', prostitutes and independent urban women adopted cosmetics as a badge of their identity in the years immediately preceding the Second World War. At the same time, men targeted cosmetic use as the symbolic attribute of 'dangerous' femininity and as an expression of their fears about women's mobility and women's power.[96] Some of the interviewed nurses noted that the heavy use of cosmetics would make them appear cheap and look like prostitutes. However, their ability to buy cosmetics and use their hard-earned money in the way they deemed fit, displayed their economic power and was a statement of their independence.

Nurses were also pacesetters concerning other social practices of the period. The use of cosmetics and trendy fashion went hand in hand with the way they spent their leisure time, as especially noted in their ballroom-dancing activities, which acted as an important testimony of their new status. *The Africa Parade* of February 1959 described the 1958 Impilo Hospital Nurses' Christmas Ball as follows:

> The Impilo Hospital Nurses' Christmas Ball was a most lovely party. Ladies swayed and swaggered in the best of dresses and the outpatients' hall was graced with both distinguished men and women of the city and galaxies of beauty. It was one of the dressiest parties the township had ever had.[97]

The leisure time affirmed female African nurses' entry into the middle class during a time of rapid economic change. Ballroom dancing was popular amongst the middle class and those who aspired to be associated with this class. Fashion was as also a marker of difference as it differentiated the older and younger generations. It also distinguished the urban from the rural and separated those who were aspiring to be part of the middle class as opposed to the urban working class. Young women used their financial power to assert their independence from the dictates of their parents' generation. The statement 'I bought clothes, I bought shoes', punctuated most of the responses to my question about how the nurses spent part of their salaries. They had the financial wherewithal to buy fashionable clothes and, being in the cities, they risked their parents' wrath by daring to wear risqué fashions such as short dresses and high-heeled shoes, instead of knee-length dresses and tennis shoes.

Conclusion

The post-Second World War era saw significant changes to nursing services in Southern Rhodesia. Key to the transformation in nursing services of the colony was the opening up of SRN training to non-Europeans. Young African women were sent to South Africa for training as SRNs. At the same time, the government began training the first cohorts of non-European nurses at Princess Margaret, Harari (Gomo) and Impilo hospitals. While the entrance of non-European women into the SRN profession was in part due to policy changes in the post-Second World War era, the privileging of government's efforts tell only one side of the story. It obscures non-European nurses' agency, in the process failing to take into consideration young women's motives for choosing the profession as a preferred career option.

Drawing on oral histories allows us to explore the varied yet interrelated reasons for choosing nursing as a career, young women's perceptions of their career, young women's agency and the socio-economic mobility amongst these young women. The reason for choosing nursing even though options were limited for many young women, ranged from the attractive nature of the occupation, the aura associated with nursing, the presence of role models and economic issues. At the same time, African nurses used the above reasons as a marker of difference between themselves and other professional women such as teachers, and also with the later generation of nurses. In addition, taking up nursing as a profession enabled African women to enter into the middle class and gave them new opportunities that were not available to earlier generations. The nursing profession allowed African women to negotiate their social and economic position with their families and communities.

An emphasis of these various motives not only opened up space to explore their hopes and aspirations within the colonial environment, but for nursing history, their recollections are shown as central in the forging of the nursing identity in Rhodesia during the post-Second World War era. The forging of the nursing identity commenced as they entered nursing school and through the everyday practice of their nursing work once they became qualified SRNs, providing care and nursing their own people in Rhodesian government hospitals from the late 1950s onwards.

Notes

1 For more on the social and economic changes that took place in post-Second World War Southern Rhodesia see R. Gray, *The two nations: Aspects of the development of race relations in Rhodesia and Nyasaland* (Oxford: Oxford University Press, 1960) and I. R. Phimister, *An economic and social history of Zimbabwe: Capital accumulation and class struggle* (Cambridge: Cambridge University Press, 1988).
2 In the years before 1952, four students per year left Rhodesia for McCord Hospital. In 1953, the government increased the bursaries to ten per annum. By 1961, seventy-one African girls from Rhodesia qualified with SRN diplomas at McCord, seventeen had gained the midwifery certificate and sixty Rhodesian nurses had both diplomas. See M. Gelfand, *A service to the sick*, p. 149.
3 NAZ Annual Report on the Public Health which covers Northern Rhodesia, Nyasaland and Southern Rhodesia (1954).
4 See *Central African Journal of Medicine*, 5: 8 (1959), p. 434.
5 *Central African Journal of Medicine*, 5: 8 (1959), p. 434.
6 NAZ Annual Report on the Public Health which covers Northern Rhodesia, Nyasaland and Southern Rhodesia (1958).
7 M. Gelfand, 'Harare Hospital ('Gomo') comes of age', *Central African Journal of Medicine*, 25: 8 (1979), pp. 177–8.
8 Gelfand, 'Harare Hospital ('Gomo') comes of age', pp. 177–8.
9 Horwitz, *Baragwanath Hospital*, p. 51
10 For this work, the term 'middle class' denotes a group of Africans who used education as a bedrock strategy to rise up the socio-economic ladder. This group included nurses, teachers, religious ministers, lawyers, journalists, civil servants, and medical doctors. Nonetheless, the reality that they marked themselves as the middle and elite class does not mean that they were completely

separated from urban workers and the peasantry. For more on the development of the African middle class in Zimbabwe see M. West, *The rise of an African middle class: Colonial Zimbabwe, 1898–1965* (Bloomington: Indiana University Press, 2002).
11 See for example T. A. Barnes, 'We women worked so hard': *Gender, urbanization and social reproduction in colonial Harare, Zimbabwe, 1930–1956* (Portsmouth, NH: Heinemann, 1999).
12 Christine Mawema quoted in *The African Parade*, December 1960.
13 Christine Mawema quoted in *The African Parade*, December 1960.
14 For more on missionaries in Zimbabwe see for example Schmidt, *Peasants, traders and wives*.
15 Interviews: Mrs Jane Mushando, Sakubva Mutare, 27 April 2009; Mrs Laiza Shumba, Mabelreign, Harare, 26 October 2008; Mrs Nhamo, Mufakose Harare, 13 September 2008; Mrs Wendy Mwamuka, Dangamvura Mutare, 17 April 2009.
16 Interviews: Mrs Nhamo, Mufakose Harare, 13 September 2008; Mrs Laiza Shumba, Mabelreign Harare, 26 October 2008; Mrs Wendy Mwamuka, Dangamvura Mutare, 17 April 2009.
17 Interview: Mrs Wendy Mwamuka, Dangamvura Mutare, 17 April 2009.
18 Interview: Mr Kufa Mutoro, Mutare, 12 August 2008.
19 Interview: Mrs Jane Mushando, Sakubva Mutare, 27 April 2009.
20 Interview: Mrs Stella Munemo, Harare Hospital, 26 August 2008.
21 West, *The rise of the African middle class*, p. 49.
22 'A' (Advanced) Level is the last two years of high school.
23 By contrast, virtually 100 per cent of white children completed secondary school with about 23 per cent going on to 'A' level. See for example A. K. H. Weinrich, *Black and white rural elites in Rhodesia* (Manchester: Manchester University Press, 1973), p. 103, and J. Pape, 'Changing education for majority rule in Zimbabwe and South Africa', *Comparative Education Review*, 42: 3 (1998), pp. 253–66.
24 The Wayfarer movement functioned in the same way as the Boy Scout movement.
25 Schmidt, *Peasants, traders and wives*, pp. 151–4.
26 Schmidt, *Peasants, traders and wives*, pp. 151–4.
27 Schmidt, *Peasants, traders and wives*, pp. 151–4.
28 Schmidt, *Peasants, traders and wives*, pp. 151–4.
29 Interview: Mrs Stella Munemo, Harare Hospital, 26 August 2008.
30 Interview: Mrs Christina Banda, Norton, July 2009.
31 Interview: Mrs Christina Banda, Norton, July 2009.
32 Interview: Mrs Nomsa Makoni, Chitungwiza, 20 April 2009.
33 Interview: Mrs Nomsa Makoni, Chitungwiza, 20 April 2009.
34 Interview: Ms Tsitsi Chinamasa, Old Mutare Mission, 28 May 2009.
35 Horwitz, *Baragwanath Hospital*, p. 132.

36 See for example, A. McClintock, *Imperial leather: Race, gender and sexuality in Colonial Conquest* (New York: Routledge, 1995).
37 T. Burke, *Lifebuoy men, Lux women: Commodification, consumption and cleanliness in modern Zimbabwe* (London: Routledge and Kegan Paul, 1996).
38 Burke, *Lifebuoy men, Lux women*.
39 Horwitz, *Baragwanath Hospital*, p. 133.
40 Interview: Mrs Nomsa Makoni, Chitungwiza, 20 April 2009.
41 Interview: Mrs Nelia Ncube, Chitungwiza, 20 April 2009.
42 Interview: Ms Esther Mawoyo, Chikanga Mutare, 22 February 2009.
43 J. Craik, *Uniforms exposed: From conformity to transgression* (Oxford, New York: Berg, 2005), p. 127.
44 Craik, *Uniforms exposed: From conformity to transgression*, p. 127.
45 Shula Marks, *Divided sisterhood*. Chapter 8.
46 Interview: Ms Esther Mawoyo, Chikanga Mutare, 22 February 2009.
47 Shula Marks, *Divided sisterhood*. Chapter 8.
48 Interviews: Mrs Jane Mushando, Sakubva Mutare, 27 April 2009, Mrs Laiza Shumba, Mabelreign Harare, 26 October 2008.
49 Interview: Mrs Jane Mushando, Sakubva Mutare, 27 April 2009.
50 Interview: Mrs Jane Mushando, Sakubva Mutare, 27 April 2009.
51 Interview: Mrs Laiza Shumba, Mabelreign Harare, 26 October 2008.
52 Interview: Mrs Laiza Shumba, Mabelreign Harare, 26 October 2008.
53 Interview: Mrs Maidei Madziwa, Sakubva Mutare, 10 February 2009.
54 Interview: Ms Esther Mawoyo, Chikanga Mutare, 22 February 2009.
55 See Chapter 6 for a full discussion of these changes.
56 Interview: Mrs Jane Mushando, Sakubva Mutare, 27 April 2009.
57 Interview: Ms Tsitsi Chinamasa, Old Mutare Mission, 28 May 2009.
58 Interview: Mrs Shumba, Mabelreign Harare, 26 October 2008.
59 African women in colonial Africa have always used the recourse of the law to redress problems and assert their independence. For example, Richard Roberts successfully demonstrated how Africans in French Soudan began seeking recourse to colonial courts to resolve their most intimate domestic disputes at the turn of the century. The use of legal routes exposed tension within African communities and at the same time provided a lens into the social and economic changes that were taking place or being accelerated by colonialism. Zimbabwean scholars have also shown how women used courts to redress injustice. See for example, R. Roberts, *Litigants and households: African disputes and colonial courts in the French Soudan, 1895–1912* (Portsmouth, NH: Heinemann, 2005); K. Benson and J. M. Chadya, 'Ukubhinya: gender and sexual violence in Bulawayo, colonial Zimbabwe, 1946-1956', *Journal of Southern African Studies*, 31: 3 (2005), pp. 587-610; and T. B. Zimudzi, 'African women, violent crime and the criminal law in Colonial Zimbabwe, 1900–1952', *Journal of Southern African Studies*, 30: 3 (2004), pp. 499–517.

60 I doubt it very much that 'other' women, usually categorised as 'low classes', would have taken such a bold step against the colonial authority.
61 During the Second World War, the British Royal Air Force had training bases in Salisbury and Gwelo. It is possible that some British officers did not strictly follow the racially inscribed policies.
62 The Location bylaws indicated that non-residents were not supposed to be in the location for more than twelve hours without the approval of the Location Superintendent.
63 NAZ LG 12/7/29. Resident Location Nurses. Entry into their quarters. 6 October 1944–18 March 1946.
64 NAZ LG 12/7/29. Resident Location Nurses. Entry into their quarters. 6 October 1944–18 March 1946. At this meeting, the Superintendent of the Location admitted that the raid had been made as the result of a report regarding harbouring of Europeans, but refused to divulge the nature or origin of the report. He also refused to either withdraw the allegations or admit that they were unfounded.
65 NAZ LG 12/7/29. Resident Location Nurses. Entry into their quarters. 6 October 1944–18 March 1946.
66 NAZ LG 12/7/29. Resident Location Nurses. Entry into their quarters. 6 October 1944–18 March 1946.
67 NAZ LG 12/7/29. Resident Location Nurses. Entry into their quarters. 6 October 1944–18 March 1946.
68 NAZ LG 12/7/29. Resident Location Nurses. Entry into their quarters. 6 October 1944–18 March 1946.
69 NAZ LG 12/7/29. Resident Location Nurses. Entry into their quarters. 6 October 1944–18 March 1946.
70 Barnes in 'We women worked so hard' noted that local governments continued to infringe upon Africans' privacy in a general and women's privacy in particular during the colonial period.
71 Y. Vera, *Butterfly burning* (Harare: Baobab Books, 1998), p. 59.
72 Interview: Mbuya Phaina Nyanhanda, Harare, 15 August 2007. Interview by P. Mukwambo.
73 Barnes, 'We women worked so hard', p. 36.
74 *The African Parade*, June 1954.
75 See for example Allison Shutt's discussion on the anti-colour bar campaigns and the struggles over desegregation of swimming pools. A. K. Shutt, *Manners make a nation: Racial etiquette in Southern Rhodesia, 1910–1963* (Rochester, NY: University of Rochester Press, 2015), pp. 149–56.
76 Michael West, *The rise of the African middle class*, p. 49.
77 Sheeben queens were women who brewed and sold liquor illegally in urban areas.
78 *The African Parade,* November 1958.
79 Interview: Mrs Christina Banda, Norton, July 2009.
80 This issue is discussed in Chapter 4.

Taking up nursing as a career, 1950–60s

81 Interview: Mrs Christina Banda, Norton, July 2009.
82 Interview: Mrs Nelia Ncube, Chitungwiza, 20 April 2009.
83 Interview: Mrs Phaina Nyanhanda, Harare, 15 August 2007. Interview by P. Mukwambo.
84 *The African Parade,* June 1957. For South Africa, see also S. Horwitz, '"Black nurses in white": Exploring young women's entry into the nursing profession at Baragwanath Hospital, Soweto, 1948–1980', *Social History Medicine,* 20: 1 (2007), pp. 131–46.
85 Interview: Mrs Mukono, Mabelreign Harare, 27 October 2008.
86 Interview: Mrs Phaina Nyanhanda, Harare, 15 August 2007. Interview by P. Mukwambo.
87 S. B. Stichter, 'The middle-class family in Kenya: Changes in gender relations', in S. B. Stichter and J. Parpart (eds), *Patriarchy and class: African women in the home and workplace* (Boulder, CO: Westview Press, 1995), pp. 177–203.
88 Interview: Mrs Phaina Nyanhanda, Harare, 15 August 2007. Interview by P. Mukwambo.
89 My informants did not remember how much they paid their maids though they claimed that it was reasonable.
90 Interview: Mrs Phaina Nyanhanda, Harare, 15 August 2007. Interview by P. Mukwambo.
91 For more, see J. Pape, 'Still serving the tea: Domestic workers in Zimbabwe 1980', *Journal of Southern African Studies,* 19: 3 (1993), pp. 387–404.
92 Interview: Mrs Laiza Shumba, Mabelreign Harare, 26 October 2008.
93 Interview: Mrs Laiza Shumba, Mabelreign Harare, 26 October 2008.
94 Interview: Mrs Maida Tsopora, Harare, 28 October 2008.
95 A. K. H. Weinrick, quoted in Burke, *Lifebuoy men, Lux women,* p. 200.
96 Burke, *Lifebuoy men, Lux women,* pp. 194–7.
97 *The African Parade,* February 1959.

4

The Africanisation of Rhodesia's clinical spaces and an anatomy of everyday work in hospitals, 1960–70

Introduction

Nursing services in Rhodesia's government hospitals in the post-Second World War period experienced a gradual and steady transformation. As previously noted, the government began opening up formal training of nursing to African women who embraced the opportunity for various reasons. These women became the backbone of nursing services, nursing their own people in government hospitals in the 1960s. This transformation, which I call the Africanisation of the hospital, began in the mid-1940s. Again, as highlighted, the baby steps of this Africanisation process can be traced back to 1945 when the government commenced with the formal training of female nurse aides at Makumbi Hospital and the midwives at Umtali Hospital. These two schemes kick-started the government's formal training of female hospital workers. Further steps were taken in the 1950s by sending young African women to South Africa, especially to McCord Hospital in Natal, and by opening the first training scheme for coloureds and people of Asian origin at Princess Margaret Hospital in 1953. Five years later, in 1958, the opening of the Impilo Hospital Nursing School and the Harari Hospital Nursing School pushed the Africanisation into full swing. It must be pointed out that the Africanisation process not only meant having formally trained African nurses within hospitals, it also led to the promotion of some of these African nurses to senior ranks within the Rhodesian Nursing Service. By appointing African nursing tutors and sisters into more senior positions, the government began the gradual dismantling of the industrial colour bar system that denied Africans positions of power within the Civil Service. Still, as will become clear, racism within hospitals continued into the late 1970s. What follows, therefore, is the story of this transformation – the Africanisation of the government hospital system in Rhodesia and its implications for African nursing staff.

Although the government began the Africanisation process, the hospital remained quintessentially a colonial space, as the hierarchy of authority and the use of power within clinical spaces replicated colonial race and class relations. An examination of student nurses' experiences – when they began the journey into nursing, expose how they traded one form of patriarchal control with another. While this was the case, experiences within nursing schools began the process of transformation from being a student nurse to a fully qualified nurse. It also started the struggle for personal independence together with African nurses' struggle to transform hospital spaces, carving out a niche for themselves and in the process making their workspaces (hospitals) their own. I thus argue that the Africanisation was not merely based on increasing the numbers of African nurses in hospitals. In addition, it was also not the mere appointing of Africans into senior positions. Africanisation was also about taking control of hospital spaces, and transforming such spaces in relation to the nature of the patient, in this case the African patient. Central to this version of Africanisation of the hospital system was the everyday nursing work done by African nurses who became the backbone of nursing services in Rhodesia from the 1960s onwards. By focusing on work and connecting it with the idea of the Africanisation of the hospital, one is able to open up space to examine the various ways in which daily nursing work is used to transform the hospital. In other words, African nurses made the colonial hospital more receptive to the African way of conduct when it came to matters dealing with illness and nursing the infirm.

At the same time, nurses' testimonies suggest that nursing practice within colonial hospitals gave African women an opportunity to reshape cultural perceptions of nursing and the care economy. It is a truism that nursing students did not arrive at the nursing school as empty vessels, devoid of values, attitudes and beliefs. They carried into their profession a constellation of the cultural values of their family, class, race and religious origins. Hence, as much as their training emphasised western medicine, African female nurses were not wholly midwives of western medicine; they drew upon their cultural norms of health and healing. Co-opting cultural understandings of therapy in hospitals enabled African nurses to come to terms with the intricacies of colonial medicine, simultaneously reformulating their own and patients' ideas of healing. At the same time, hospital work enabled African women to push the cultural boundaries of nursing. An anatomy of their stories of encounters with strangers' bodies, elderly patients and dead bodies gives us an understanding of the various ways in which African women came to terms with new forms of healing at the same time as providing insight into how they remoulded their culturally specific African nursing practices.

The Africanisation of Rhodesian clinical spaces

To understand the complexities of workplace culture during the period under study, it is necessary to briefly examine the racial changes that took place within nursing services from the post-Second World War era onwards. By the end of the war, Rhodesian authorities began laying the groundwork for African trained nurses to work in government hospitals. With an anticipated 'increase in birth rates' and the expected 'massive development of general medical maternity services',[1] the African midwife became the immediate focus for government policy. The birthplace for the midwifery programme was at the Umtali African Midwives Government School, with a cohort of six students. Just as missionaries had earlier done with young African women at mission stations, government midwifery training emphasised western medical intricacies. At the same time, the government expected the midwives to convince African women of the ostensible advantages of maternity clinics in the colony.[2] As Laiza Shumba noted when reflecting on the burden placed on African midwives: 'Our elder sisters who worked at mission hospitals and those trained by the government as midwives preached the gospel of cleanliness and coaxed more African women to give birth in hospitals.'[3] The government considered the pilot programme at Umtali a considerable success to the extent that it adopted an expanded and modified version of the programme for the Harari and Bulawayo African hospitals. The government also increased student intake from six to twelve students per cohort. The quest for better-qualified midwives saw an extension of the apprenticeship years from one to two.[4] These midwives became the cornerstone of maternity clinics in African urban and rural areas.

Government midwifery training presented an opportunity for African women to highlight their potential and make significant contributions to the Rhodesian healthcare system. At the same time, African midwives' training provides us an opportunity to analyse the government's attitude towards Africans in general and African women in particular. Specifically, it showed the government's recognition of the importance of African women's service to the hospital system by the beginning of the second half of the century. Furthermore, it was also an acknowledgment of and a testament to African women's knowledge and skill within birthing spaces. When African women officially entered colonial birthing spaces as government-employed midwives, they relieved European midwives of the supposed burden of nursing African maternity patients. It quickly became clear that they served only one section of the African population, given that their training focused on mothers and infants. Thus, already short of trained nurses,[5] it was critical on the part of the authorities to train African women as State Registered Nurses (SRNs) for the rest of the patient population. In the long term, the training of SRNs shifted the burden of nursing African patients from European nurses. Consequently, it freed European nurses from concentrating on African patients and enabled them to focus on European patients.

The training of SRNs presented a significant challenge to policy and the colonial system. In a quest to 'uphold nursing standards' and uniformity, authorities required that health officials teach the same curriculum across races. The SRN course took forty-eight months to complete. It had a greater emphasis on theory although clinical practice was also significant. Furthermore, the SRN course had to be taught at hospitals with more than fifty beds to give students experiences with diverse medical problems.[6] At a time when segregation was the pillar of society, the Rhodesian government had to provide nursing schools to Africans. Yet, until 1958 when the government's Impilo and Harari hospitals began functioning, training schools for African SRNs in Rhodesia were conspicuous by their absence. The government was in a dilemma. The lack of government African training schools until 1958 meant that to train African SRNs, authorities had to open up well-equipped European hospitals and training schools for African nursing candidates. Such an undertaking would inevitably undermine the backbone of Rhodesian racial policy: the colour-bar system and racial separation. Furthermore, if African nursing students were allowed to train in European nursing schools, this gesture would have blurred and eventually set in motion the erosion of racial boundaries within clinical spaces.[7]

The case of the coloured and Asian communities further illuminates the use of clinical spaces by Rhodesian authorities to enforce the philosophy of racial separation and segregation. Following this principle, the government expected African nurses to work in African hospitals only, and in African wards of government hospitals in smaller towns. Structurally, however, colonial society had three racial hierarchies: Europeans, coloured/Asians and Africans, in that order. There was also a need, therefore, for government to train coloured and Asian SRNs to work in Asian and coloured wards. In the late 1940s, the Asian and coloured communities petitioned the government to build a hospital for their community. Their victory came in 1952. In line with its policy of total segregation based on colour, the government established the Princess Margaret Hospital in Salisbury for coloureds and Asians. Besides concentrating on the coloured/Asian patient, the hospital also focused on training Asian/coloured young women. Thus, in 1953, the government started training coloured and Asian nursing students. This group was the pioneer cohort of non-Europeans to qualify as SRNs in Rhodesia.[8] By policy, Asian/coloured nurses were only supposed to be trained in their hospitals. However, when faced with problems, authorities ignored policy, even though they tried to avoid upsetting European patients over this arrangement. Again, the case of Asian/coloured students in Bulawayo illustrates this point. In 1960, the government suggested the possibility of having coloured/Asian trainee nurses conduct part of their practical training in the European hospital. As Bulawayo had a smaller number of coloured/Asian nursing students,[9] the authorities hoped to curb the inefficiency of having tutors teach practical nursing to two groups, whites and Asians/coloureds separately. After raising the issue with matrons and sister tutors and discussing the matter with trained European nursing staff, the Medical Superintendent of Bulawayo Central Hospital felt that it was a possibility since there were hardly any complaints about the matter. Part of the letter read:

> They [white nurses] felt that in principle there is no objection to coloured and Asian student nurses doing their practicals in European wards. But they felt that from time to time there would be occasional clashes with certain patients. We further discussed this at the Hospital Advisory Committee and the members all agreed to the principle, but they realised that there would be occasional difficulties with certain patients. It was agreed that Coloured and Asiatic (Asian) student nurses could be introduced into the Central Hospital and that every effort would be made by the staff to avoid personality clashes.[10]

The fear of antagonising white patients was still prevalent. However, for practical reasons, hospital authorities at times ignored the rule, though maintaining the distance between white patients and coloured/Asian trainee nurses. In 1961, the Secretary for Health confirmed that coloured and Asian student nurses in Bulawayo could conduct part of their practical nurse training at the European Central Hospital.[11] This was merely an exception to the rule to student nurses in the early 1960s. Authorities maintained that white nurses were the only suitable nurses to nurse white patients. In the same letter to the Director of Medical Service, the Medical Superintendent of Bulawayo Central Hospital dismissed the idea of having trained Asian/coloured nurses practice their craft in white hospitals and white wards: 'it has further been suggested that coloured and Asian staff might be used in the Central Hospital. This would, I think lead to greater difficulties at this stage.'[12] It was not until the late 1960s, faced with problems of staffing white wards, that the government began allowing a few coloured and Asian State Registered Nurses to work in white wards. Important to appreciate is that they worked under white nurses' supervision.

Opening up European or Asian/coloured hospitals to young African women would have eroded the racial boundaries that authorities had tried hard to maintain. What happened between the end of the Second World War and 1958 when the government opened Harari and Impilo hospitals to young African women to train as SRNs demonstrated the efforts by Rhodesian authorities to maintain racial separation in clinical spaces. To circumvent this predicament of training young African women with other races, the government looked for assistance from its most trusted neighbour across the Limpopo River. Rhodesian authorities turned to South Africa for help to train SRNs at least until they had completed building African hospitals with the capacity and equipment to train African SRNs.[13] Hence, by the beginning of the 1950s, the Ministry of Health began offering young African women bursaries to train as SRNs in South Africa. McCord Hospital, in present-day KwaZulu-Natal, became one of the leading destinations for trainee nurses. Initially, four students per year left Rhodesia for McCord Hospital. In 1953, the government increased the bursaries to ten per annum. By 1961, seventy-one young African women from Rhodesia qualified with SRN diplomas from McCord, seventeen had gained the midwifery certificate, and sixty had obtained both diplomas.[14] These African nurses came back home to serve their people. While the government was sending students abroad, in 1958 the first cohort of government-trained African nurses started their courses at Impilo Hospital in Bulawayo and Harari Hospital. These young women together with their counterparts trained abroad, changed the structure of nursing services in Rhodesia. The African State Registered Nurse had finally come home (Figure 4.1).

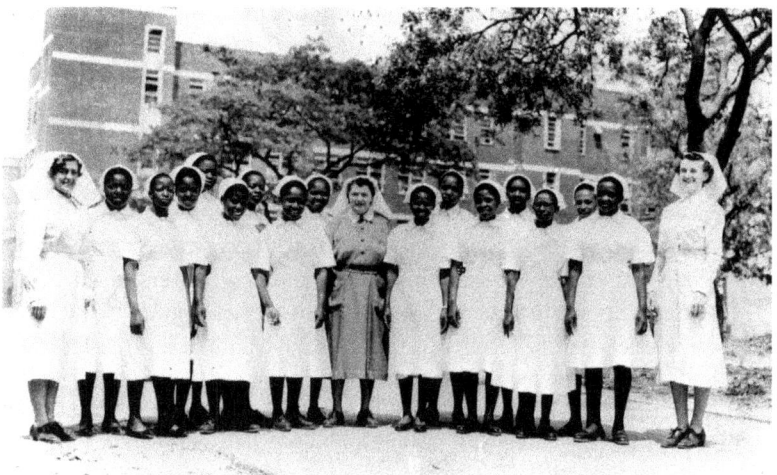

Figure 4.1 Harare Hospital trainees (195-) [Date incomplete] (courtesy National Archives of Zimbabwe)

National politics played an important part in influencing the transformations, namely, the Africanisation of nursing services during the time under discussion. From 1953 to 1963, Southern Rhodesia was part of the Federation of Rhodesia and Nyasaland.[15] A key aspect of the Federation was the 'partnership' concept. For Europeans, partnership was a socio-political system based on the maintenance of racial identity and political and economic cooperation between races. In practice, racial segregation was the fulcrum of the policy, with Europeans in control as the senior partners in the arrangement.[16] Africans thought otherwise. According to African nationalist Bernard Chidzero, by 'partnership' Africans meant 'equality of individuals before the law, regardless of race or colour'. It denoted a political and social system based on persons rather than groups. Specifically, it meant 'the total abolition of discrimination on the grounds of race'.[17] Regarding employment, Colin Leys noted that Southern Rhodesia amended the Industrial Conciliation Act of 1958, enabling Africans to join Trade Unions. Thus the Trade Unions could be multiracial, and concerning the Civil Service, in 1959, Southern Rhodesia altered the Civil Service Act, which had in effect excluded African Civil Servants from the rights and privileges accorded to white Civil Servants. Writing in 1960, Colin Leys noted:

> The Federal Public Service regulations permit Africans to hold jobs in the highest pay scales ... African nurses are being trained by the Department of Health and will be able to earn European salaries if they qualify.[18]

While Leys was optimistic over the possibilities of the government's gradual dismantling of racialised salary structures within the Civil Service, this never took place. As my informants suggested, one's race determined the salary earned. The government paid experienced and qualified African nurses lower salaries in comparison to their European counterparts.[19]

The Federation of Rhodesia and Nyasaland brought new opportunities for many. Likewise, the introduction of the Federal Civil Service in 1953 and its subsequent expansion to cater for the Federation's needs was also reflected in clinical spaces as government created new posts for European nurses. The building of African hospitals also created openings for African nurses. The potential offered by the Federation made it possible for African nurses to imagine moving up the civil service ladder. Realising that it was impractical and impossible to rely solely on European women with all responsibilities related to African wards, the government began opening up important posts to African nurses. Before 1961, the government placed all African nurses in Branch III of the Federal Nursing Services. This was one of the lowest grades within the Civil Service. Based on racial hierarchy, the grading system failed to take educational qualifications into consideration and deliberately ignored skill and seniority.[20] By the end of 1960, changes for African nurses were in the air. In January 1961, the government upgraded twenty-five nurses, twenty-one from Impilo Hospital in Bulawayo and four from Harari Hospital into the Branch II of the Federal Nursing Service structure. Branch II of the Federal Nursing Service, which was also part of Branch II of the Civil Service structure, was created as a proving ground for 'non-Europeans who, for reasons both of their qualifications and of the duties they are performing, can, provided they exhibit the necessary qualities of character, merit advancement to Branch I on parity with European officers'.[21] Promotion into Branch II did not automatically mean that African nurses were on par with their European counterparts. They had to prove themselves, as per policy, before they could qualify for Branch I. This was in direct contrast to their European counterparts, who, because of their race, automatically entered Branch I of the Federal Nursing Service. Thus, as much as there were changes within the Civil Service structure, African women remained under the tutelage of their European counterparts.[22] As Flora Matondo recalled, 'There were many disparities during the colonial period. We were under whites who treated us as servants no matter one's qualifications. Young white nurses had more power than us. They could give you instructions on what to do. Even if I knew I was qualified, there was nothing I could do about that, we had to do our work.'[23] Discrimination in the workplace was rife, and this frustrated many African nurses. The partnership remained unequal. Nevertheless, promotions were a major step for African nurses and recognition of African women's service to their people.

The promotion of nurses was met with mixed feelings by African nurses. Evidence suggests that such a step that recognised their competence in an environment that circumscribed upward mobility for African women, elated the nurses.[24] Laiza Shumba remembered how, as a student nurse, her cohort looked up to these women who had moved up the ladder as role models and people who inspired them to succeed in life. According to her, 'They had shown us that we could as Africans improve our position if we want. It was a testimony of good things to come for nurses.'[25] This upward mobility gave nurses hope. They were ecstatic over the possibilities offered to them. However, nurses at Harari Hospital bitterly complained about what they saw as unfair treatment of Harari nurses as compared to nurses at Impilo in Bulawayo. The nursing authorities upgraded only four nurses from Harari as compared to twenty-one from Impilo. Though direct evidence is lacking, one can speculate that African nurses complained to their authorities at Harari Hospital, and clear evidence of the disgruntlement comes from an editorial in *The African Weekly*. In part, it read:

> If African State Registered Nurses at Harari Hospital are genuinely working hard for their hospital to be the best in the Federation, they have cause to be bitterly disappointed with the recent upgrading published in our last week's issue. The upgrading of only four of their hospital staff – compared to 21 at Impilo – has knocked down to zero the prestige of their hospital. And because the upgrading is supposed to depend on efficiency, it has suggested that Harari is packed with inefficient nurses. We challenge health authorities to deny this or otherwise to confirm it and state if it is by coincidence.[26]

Oral interviews and archival sources were vague on whether there was a struggle and rivalry between Harari and Impilo hospitals. In addition, sources were unclear whether this struggle, if it existed, was due to ethnic differences or a reflection of the struggles between Salisbury and Bulawayo as major urban centres in Rhodesia. Nevertheless, from the complaints in newspapers, one can detect that nurses at Harari felt unfairly treated. Harari Hospital nurses petitioned the government to upgrade more senior nurses from their institution. The pressure worked as the government immediately took steps to remedy the problem. It appointed sixteen more nurses by mid-January of the same year, of which fifteen were from Harari Hospital.[27] These promotions were a crucial step in the restructuring of the Nursing Service that ultimately saw African women taking up greater responsibilities in hospitals.

The changes went beyond appointing African SRNs into Branch II of the Federal Nursing Service. The government began promoting non-European nurses to higher and more influential ranks. There is no evidence indicating that before 1962, Rhodesia had African or coloured nursing sisters or nursing tutors. While African and coloured SRNs were still few, the policy that placed African and coloured nurses into Branch II of the Nursing Service and white nurses into Branch I made it easy to overlook and side-line African and coloured nurses. Younger and less experienced white nurses had a higher chance of promotion in comparison to African and coloured nurses.[28] The year 1962 saw another significant policy shift. On 1 June 1962, Charity Munjoma became the first African SRN to be promoted to the rank of sister in the Federal Government Service.[29] Working at Lusaka Central Hospital, Munjoma was one of the many African nurses who studied nursing in South Africa. A graduate of McCord Hospital, Munjoma had been in government employ for fourteen years. Due to government policy, she was employed first as a nursing assistant and later as junior nurse even though she was fully qualified.

In addition, irrespective of her impressive educational qualifications, Munjoma worked under the supervision of European nurses. It was only with the inception of the Federation that government recognised nurses of her calibre as SRNs. Thus, Munjoma's appointment as the first African nursing sister represented another significant milestone in African women's advancement within the Nursing Service. At the time of her appointment and in the months immediately following, the government expected to assign more experienced non-European nurses to the position of sisters. The government appointed four more nursing sisters in 1962 to make it a total of five.[30] Important to note is that the government posted three of the five nursing sisters to hospitals outside Southern Rhodesia. Munjoma and Nhlahla found themselves at Lusaka Central Hospital in Northern Rhodesia, while the government posted Sondo to Blantyre Hospital in Nyasaland. The two other non-European nurses, both coloured nurses, were stationed in Southern Rhodesia.[31] As part of the Federal policy, nurses could be posted anywhere within the Federation. It is highly likely that vacancies for African nurses to work in senior positions were available in Lusaka and Blantyre. The year 1963 saw the dismantling of the Federation, and the Rhodesian Front declared Rhodesia independent from Britain in 1964. The policy of Africanising the nursing services continued. The late 1960s had more Africans in positions of influence in Southern Rhodesia than before. In fact, by the end of the 1960s and into the early 1970s, African hospitals were more Africanised. Informants indicated that there were African nursing tutors, matrons and sisters in charge of wards in African hospitals.[32]

The world of the student nurse and the struggle for independence

Nursing school played a significant role in the transformation of young African women. It must be noted that by entering nursing school, young African women were moving away from the daily patriarchal control in their homes to another version of control.[33] This was not a novel phenomenon amongst African women in Rhodesia. At the turn of the nineteenth and twentieth centuries, young African women ran away to mission stations in search of independence.[34] Although later generations of young African women in the 1950s and 1960s sought parental blessing to enter nursing school, like their grandmothers, they perceived nursing school as an avenue towards independence from male guardians.[35] Just like young women who fled to mission stations in the years around 1900, trainee nurses later in the twentieth century traded one form of patriarchal control for another. Their stories bring to the fore nursing students' continued experience under new forms of paternalistic relationships and their struggles for social independence. The struggles with matrons to assert their autonomy punctuated the experiences of many.

During the 1950s and 1960s, the typical hospital structure reflected colonial racial structures. White men, administrators and medical doctors occupied the top of the pyramid while an army of African workers occupied the base. In between were white matrons, sisters and nursing tutors. White matrons and sister tutors wielded formidable power. They managed a staff of white nurses and African hospital workers upon which they exerted tight control. They directed a wide range of clinical, domestic and administrative tasks. Just below the powerful white matriarchs were sisters, junior nurses and temporarily employed European nurses who also wielded a lot of authority over black nurses. Younger and inexperienced white nurses at times supervised African nurses.[36] There were slight changes by the end of the 1960s and into the 1970s as more Africans occupied senior positions within African hospitals. This did not drastically change the relationship between senior nurses and junior nurses. As Sekai Nzenza described in her semi-autobiographical *Zimbabwean Woman: My Own Story*, African nursing tutors and sisters replicated an inherited hierarchy of order and authority. They were as strict with nursing students as were white matrons, sisters and tutors. According to Nzenza, 'African nursing sisters and tutors were nothing short of black women, living and behaving like white women ... a nursing student could be dismissed for a minor malfeasance without warning.'[37] Her ordeal under a black nursing sister for what she claimed was a minor misdemeanour was a testament to how both white and African nursing leaders maintained authority over nursing students:

> All day I scrubbed and polished the wheels of the trolley. I wheeled each one of them into the office for her inspection. She moved the trolley by pushing it with her leg, it made a squeaking noise. She said it was not clean and I had to do it again. I oiled all the wheels, so that they did not make any more squeaking noises. This did not make things any different. At the end of six weeks, she gave me a report. I got a *D* which meant *very poor, lazy and uncooperative*. I was sent to the white, big chested matron. She warned me that another report like this one would warrant my dismissal. I promised to co-operate and I did co-operate. I never said no to any Sister, and I worked very hard to impress them.[38]

Many an informant alluded to this strict disciplinary environment within the hospitals. Irrespective of their race, the seniors were bent on making sure that they got the best out of their students, and they would not tolerate misdemeanours as hospital authorities gave greater power to matrons and sisters over student nurses.

African student nurses' experiences within Rhodesian hospitals were not peculiar. Nurses in other parts of the world had similar experiences in their transitions towards fully-fledged nurses. The hospital was a school, workplace and home combined. As Barbara Melosh argued in the case of the United States, to initiate young women into a common occupational identity, hard work and strict discipline were emphasised.[39] Similarly, in Rhodesia, hospital officials and senior nursing personnel applied such principles to African nursing students. Matrons and sisters ensured their control over nursing students' daily work and their social lives. Their authority extended beyond the normal limits of school or workplace discipline. According to Phaina Nyanhanda,

> We began as twenty-seven and by the time we finished we were eleven. Of course, two left just after our first post mortem experience and they were very strict, especially the tutors. They had strict rules maybe because of us being black. If you make some complains, either related to food or something, they will weed out the ringleaders or either discipline them but in most cases they were expelled. We were not allowed much social interaction. If you sneaked to a local teacher's college, you will be given a stern warning and continued malfeasance will result in your dismissal from the programme. In addition, as first year students they would never tolerate mistakes with prescriptions.[40]

Her contemporary, Laiza Shumba, also stressed the sternness of the matrons and sisters in her nursing school reminiscences:

> The rules were firmer than what we have today. Young women these days have it easy. It was difficult for us to leave nursing grounds without permission. Our boyfriends were not allowed near nursing homes. We were told that we could not combine marriage with school. We had to be dedicated with our work.[41]

The emphasis on differences between the earlier generation and present-day generation was important for many older nurses. Besides exposing generational differences between older nurses and younger nurses, it was an affirmation of older nurses' suitability for the job, their dedication to serving their people and the way in which the strictness of matrons and authorities moulded them into better nurses.[42] Curfews 'protected' African nursing students from the 'prying African men'.[43] They were also an attempt to control student nurses' movements and limit their interactions with the outside world. This was aimed at making sure they concentrated on their nursing.

It is tempting to view nursing schools as 'total institutions' that imposed rigid discipline on nursing students' lives. True, their lives were regimented and organised in a hierarchy. However, training schools were not 'total institutions' as nursing students found various ways in which to circumvent these restrictions. A 1961 letter to *The African Weekly* suggested that nurses, 'misbehave with their boyfriends, are lazy (they) do not know how to keep their homes clean, nurses worry about money and getting married to rich people and so on.'[44] Cephas Msipa's memoir suggested that Harari Hospital was a destination for potential suitors. A teacher and later on, a nationalist, Msipa bought a car and drove to Harari Hospital even though he did not possess a driver's licence. He wrote, 'In those days, State Registered Nurses earned more than teachers and looked down on us, calling us "pedestrians" who couldn't afford their own transport. I had driven to Harari Hospital to show them that I had graduated from being a pedestrian to be an owner of a car.'[45] Such visits to Harari Hospital might have been popular amongst Salisbury's black male elite. *The African Weekly* captured what the African population in Salisbury thought:

> All is not well at Harari Hospital. Repeatedly, we hear stories of discord. The girls (young women) in training do not seem to have anybody looking after them. They wander with boys around hospital. Some of then spend nights out and one by one, they are being expelled as expectant mothers. This is not the way the now qualified nurses were looked after whilst in training in the Union or we should not be having one of them here. Can the Health Department sincerely tell us that there is nothing they can do to rectify things at the Harari Hospital? Or do they honestly believe there is nothing to rectify there? If so, may we be told exactly what is happening at this hospital.[46]

In response to these reports, authorities tightened their boarding regulations for trainee nurses. Thus, in July 1961, *The African Weekly* reported that:

> It has been learnt that the freedom allowed student nurses at Harari to receive visitors is even more restricted than announced in the *African Weekly* last week. They are allowed to have visitors only two days a week on Fridays and Sundays. They can have friends and relatives visit them on Fridays from 6 pm to 8 pm and on Sundays from 3 pm to 6 pm. The girls (young women) are not allowed to have visitors any other time.[47]

Such toughness on nursing students was based on a paternalistic attitude that infantilised them. Racial changes within the nursing leadership did not alter this view. As Nzenza illustrated, 'They all wanted to be the first to discover a pregnant student nurse. Pregnancy meant immediate dismissal. The matron even went to the extent of going to the nearest Family Planning Centre to find out which student nurse was registered on the pill.'[48] It is possible that the yearly average of pregnancy among nursing students was high during the colonial period. Nursing students used various coping strategies to assert their independence. Interviews suggested the prevalence of sneaking out and of nurses covering for each other. Some used their church time or what little of their leisure time to meet with their would-be partners.[49] For those who got pregnant, illegal abortion was an option if a student wanted to continue her studies.[50] In a study on abortion amongst African American women, L. J. Ross noted that abortion, in and of itself, does not automatically create freedom. However, it allowed some control over biology, freeing women from the inevitability of unwanted pregnancy. According to Ross, for those who aborted, it was necessary, as the midwife to their daily survival politics.[51] Likewise, for some of the nurses who found themselves pregnant, resorting to illegal abortion formed part of their survival politics in an effort to continue with their education.

Others turned to contraception, especially the pill and the Depo-Provera injection. According to Amy Kaler, the first use of the pill in Rhodesia was made available in 1961 to sixty white women. The provision of the pill was later extended to women of all races, so that by 1963 an estimated 3,000 doses of the pill were being sold monthly, and 'many educated women are using it, but they do not wish for it to be generally known'.[52] By 1970, the Family Planning Association reported a constant increase in the demand for the pill and the Depo-Provera injection, which in time surpassed the pill in popularity.[53] At its introduction, Africans associated the pill with promiscuity. This initial stigma made many unwilling to disclose that they were taking the pill. However, its popularity was an indicator of how African women were quick to adopt new methods of birth control in Rhodesia. For young trainee nurses who were under strict supervision from authorities, the use of contraception was part of the daily struggles to control their fertility and to assert their reproductive rights. As they were expected to teach family planning and reproductive health was part of the curriculum, nurses used their knowledge as an affirmation of their independence.[54] African women, as Kaler argued, have always used various forms of contraception as both a social and personal strategy. They used contraception in a careful and calculated way as they struggled with being good wives, good mothers and good sisters.[55] Likewise, student nurses used contraception as a personal strategy as they struggled to conform to what was expected of them as student nurses. It was part of the struggle to balance the expectations of being good student nurses and the demands of social life.

In the wards: Nurses and their everyday work

For those young African women who had the chance to enter nursing school in post-Second World War Rhodesia, their lives were fundamentally changed. As with hospital work in other parts of the world, nursing school introduced its regimented system in their lives, with trained nurses spending most of their time in class or doing practical work in wards.[56] During the first three months, nurses were under probationary training at a Preliminary Training School (PTS). Probationary training acclimatised students to the hospital system whilst simultaneously granting matrons and nurse tutors the opportunity to assess students and weed out those considered unsuitable for nursing.[57] During their initial three months at PTS, student nurses were not involved in any ward work nor night duty, but instead spent their time from 8:00 a.m. to 4:00 p.m. in class.[58] At the end of three months, students' suitability to nursing was assessed through written and oral examinations in anatomy, physiology and hygiene.[59] Thereafter, in addition to regular lectures, student nurses were transferred to a monthly basis and fulltime duty and training in hospital wards. After the first year (Preliminary Part II), nurses took written and practical examinations. Those who failed were allowed to repeat once.[60] Examiners administered the final examinations in written form, via practical assessments and *viva voce* after no less than three and a half years' training in medicine, medical nursing, surgical nursing and gynaecology nursing.[61] In short, their schedule at training over the course was three months of PTS, twenty-nine months on day duty, twelve months of night duty and four months of leave spread over the entire course.[62]

The employment of African women within government hospitals was aimed at relieving white women from the responsibility of nursing African patients. Thus, when they entered clinical spaces, African women immediately shouldered the major burden of hospital work. Work within wards increased in relation to the upsurge of patients visiting hospitals in the post-war era. The situation at the Municipal Clinic in Salisbury in 1954 gives us a glimpse of the changes that were taking place in many parts of the colony. In 1954, the Salisbury City Council complained of the increase in attendance at the Municipal Clinic's antenatal unit. According to the Medical Officer of Health, the increase not only strained Salisbury Council's medical budget but also increased nurses' workload at the clinic. To be sure, although the Municipal Clinic had an antenatal unit, this was not meant to cater to a large number of women. Only women registered to stay in the Location were the intended users of the clinic.[63] Before the opening of Harari Hospital in 1958, those not registered to stay in the Location had to use the African section of the Salisbury Hospital. However, the post-Second World War period saw major changes with more women, especially married ones moving to urban areas to stay with their husbands.[64] At the same time, it became even more difficult for the City Council to keep track of women staying in the Location. This scenario, no doubt, strained resources in African townships. As the 1954 Council Minutes indicated: 'Patient increases in the township are partly due to the rising number of married women surreptitiously taking up residence in the location.'[65] Furthermore, the clinic experienced an increase in antenatal cases from women living within the surrounding areas. By law, non-resident women living outside the Location were supposed to attend antenatal examinations at Salisbury Hospital rather than at the Location Clinic. To ease pressure on its staff, the Location Clinic refused care to non-location women and those clandestinely staying within the Location. As the Minister of Health complained of the Council's actions, women 'lead a precarious existence without any antenatal supervision and finally present themselves for admission to the Maternity hospital already in labour'.[66] This placed an added strain on the mothers and the hospital staff, which had to deal with obstetric emergencies some of which could have been pre-empted by appropriate antenatal care.

In the post-Second World War period, hospitals experienced higher increases in admissions than before. Annual patient admissions increased by almost a third from 206,514 to 324,391 between 1953 and 1959. The number of yearly outpatients attending government hospitals, clinics and dispensaries rose from an average of 1,800,000 in 1953 to 3,000,000 in the year 1959.[67] Likewise, one can speculate that mission hospitals also experienced increases during this time. While authorities claimed these increases were a result of the 'breakdown of superstition', such increases were mainly ascribed to the immigration into Rhodesia experienced in the wake of the improved economic condition. Oral sources also suggest a significant surge in the number of visitors by the mid-1950s and this no doubt led to the increase in nurses' workloads as Laiza Shumba remembered.[68] By the 1960s, as Esther Mawoyo recalled, the Casualty and Out Patient Department at Harari Hospital was always congested with patients.[69]

Even though nurses worked under so much pressure, they were more eager to talk about their work in wards as this was central in defining their professional identity. After all, their primary purpose of taking up the profession was to help the infirm and heal the sick. Their ward work, duties, the joys of nursing and the challenges they faced defined who they were and how they worked around the clock for the good of their communities. Their work varied according to the wards they worked in: whether they were assigned to the medical, general, or maternity ward, for example. Furthermore, the different times of the day they worked also had an impact on the differences in everyday work. The experienced a greater workload during the day than at night. Being a senior nurse or a junior nurse also affected the differences in work. In their first year, student nurses spent more time in classrooms than in wards. They did not shoulder the burden of ward work, as their main contribution in the wards was to help senior students and fully qualified nurses.[70] Jane Mushando remembers her training years as challenging:

> It was a lot of work as the workload was just heavy. This was coupled with the long working hours we experienced. In most cases, it left us exhausted especially when there was an emergency as we had to do a lot of running around. In most cases we worked more than 8 hours a day and the next day one had to come back early and sometime one had to switch to night duty ... We did much the same though we must acknowledge that there were cases that as first years we might not be familiar with. These we had to leave them to our seniors. For example, issues dealing with injections. As first years we were not expected to give patients injections as we were still considered as immature in the profession but there were other things that did not matter in what year one was in, we did the same, for example recording temperature, taking notes and giving medication. One thing we have to note is that at times our seniors supervised us, particularly those in third years.[71]

As student nurses, being able to conduct certain tasks was in itself a marker of difference between cohorts. A patient would be assured that an experienced student nurse would carry out intravenous injections, for example, better than a student in their first year would.[72] In addition, in their third year, many a student nurse would have gained enough knowledge and experience to work in different wards without direct supervision.[73] The normal completion time was three years, but others took a fourth year doing a midwifery course. There was a tendency amongst nursing students to specialise in working in specific clinical spaces such as the surgical ward or with specific diseases like tuberculosis. By the time they graduated, nursing students would have been exposed to the various ways in which the hospital worked, to the treatment of various diseases, and to a diverse array of patients.

Hospital administrators shuffled student nurses between wards and departments throughout the forty-eight months of training.[74] However, the most significant change to this arrangement occurred when they graduated. As junior nurses and staff nurses, they had more responsibilities and a reputation to build. Different wards required specific attention related to the nature of patients, diseases and sickness. Nurses claimed that the Out Patient Department (OPD) was the most demanding of all other hospital departments. Catering for less serious and first time patients, the OPD was organised differently to other wards. Open between 8:00 a.m. and 4:30 p.m., the OPD was central in the administration of the hospital and the patients. Documentation and paper work for patients began in the OPD. Although nurses took care of what they considered minor problems such as headaches and toothaches, for example, the presence of seriously sick patients meant that nurses had to gather more information concerning the illness. Flora Matondo highlighted that during the 1950s and 1960s:

> Many of our patients would have visited other healers. Therefore, we will ask them so that we will try to map out what exactly had been going on and what took them too long to seek medical attention at the hospital. We noticed that many people would have visited *n'angas* (traditional healers) and *vaporofita* (healers from independent African churches) and we would want to know everything. You do not know what they might have been told to take and this might have implications of our efforts to heal them.[75]

To contextualise, Shona and Ndebele cosmology identified three causes of illness: natural illness, spiritually induced illness and witchcraft.[76] In addition, when an individual was afflicted by an illness, the standard approach by Africans involved the mobilisation of a constellation of people, in what anthropologist John Janzen termed the 'therapy management group'.[77] The group was charged with the afflicted person's care.[78] This cosmology informed patients' and their relatives' understanding of illness. Africans recognised short common illnesses as a natural and normal part of life and regarded prolonged illnesses with the suspicion that someone must be the causative factor. In their study of attitudes towards illness at Harari Hospital towards the end of the colonial period, J. Kavumbura and R. T. Mossop identified three phases in processes of healing. During the first phase, the patient regarded it as natural and expected the problem to disappear within a short space of time. In the second phase, the patient sought medical help outside the home. The hospital was the next stop for patients. Prolonged hospital stays or illnesses with poor progress gave rise to self-searching and suspicion. Thus, at times relatives took the patient out of the hospital for a short time or permanently. The absence of a patient did not mean the cessation for the search for healing. Sometimes the relatives consulted the n'anga (traditional healer) without the patient.[79] While Kavumbura and Mossop presented a linear response to illness by Africans, interviews suggested that responses to illness were entangled affairs.[80] To the consternation of the hospital staff, some relatives would sneak herbs/medicine to admitted patients. According to nurses, the occurrence of such a situation complicated their work as a cocktail of medicine made it difficult to 'concentrate on the real cause of illnesses'.[81] Nurses argued that patients' failure to be clear on what had taken place during their sojourn at other healing centres frustrated them and made their work even more difficult. With the lack of documented medical history, nurses came up with other strategies to get a full picture of the nature and length of illness. According to Fadzai Mugove, 'because we did not have full documentation, we had to turn to relatives. Although information might not be necessarily accurate, at least we will try to come up with what is the best from various sources.'[82] Within African healing systems, relatives have played an important role in influencing the nature of treatment and in diagnosing.

After acquiring information needed for patient diagnosis, nurses checked the vital signs including recording temperature, blood pressure, pulse and respiration. This was the first contact with most patients. Checking vital signs, making charts and documentation, asserted nurses' independence and ascertained their importance to the hospital system.[83] While the majority of patients in the OPD were treated and sent home on the same day, nurses immediately admitted cases considered seriously ill. Nyaradzo Buzengwe reiterated that:

> Most of our admitted patients came via the OPD. In the OPD, they will have done everything for us, checking the vital signs and giving specific information to the problems affecting the patients. This was good, as it would lessen the burden of that work in the wards. However, there were also emergency cases where someone comes in and they are chronically ill or in most cases when there was an accident. We had to do everything from documentation to assigning beds and moving them to beds.[84]

It was the responsibility of orderlies to do the heavy-duty work within the wards, including transporting patients from different wards. It is important to appreciate that, even though work in the main hospital was different, depending on which wards, the nature of the patients' illness and the fact that patients changed every day, meant that one could trace a routine in nurses' work that was repeated almost every day. Nyaradzo Buzengwe remembered that:

> Every morning we started by examining files in case something might have happened during night. For example, the condition of the patient might have been more serious or someone died. We also took note of the patients who had been admitted at night. We would also prepare medication. At this time, some student nurses and orderlies will be providing food. Some patients would have taken a bath, if they can walk. For those seriously ill we would bed-bath them. Linen was changed after they had taken their food and then they are given medication. Depending on the day, the doctor will make rounds, take notes and discharge patients. By midday, we would be tired of walking up and down the wards, either making sure that everything is done properly, patients are fed, and they have taken medication. At the same time, others will be preparing the afternoon medication. We always had to be alert as there was a lot going on. The situation will become tenser when there is an emergency and we noticed more of this during the war.[85]

Nurses had preferences for in which wards they wanted to work. Tsitsi Chinamasa enjoyed working in the maternity ward more than the surgical ward, whilst Nyardzo Buzengwe enjoyed working in the OPD.[86] Most nurses stated they experienced more problems in the psychiatry and the male wards than in other wards. Even though they had these preferences, their main aim in taking up the profession was to take care of the infirm and heal the sick. Thus, they were prepared to work in any ward and such hard work, cumbersome as it was, was part of their contribution to their communities.

Nurses understood their work in a number of ways. The nature of their profession and its conduct elevated them above other professional women. Even the earliest nursing assistants, who were mainly trained to work as house cleaners, used their work to ascertain their professional superiority as compared to other women. M. Sandelowski argued, in the case of the United States, that while there were few clinical objects in the early decade of training that distinguished nurses from other women, nurses were to be distinguished from other workers by the skilful use of clinical devices such as stethoscopes and thermometers.[87] Mopping the floor, dusting and arranging flowers were part of the management of the environment around the patient. Changing bed sheets and making beds is universally part of women's work, yet nurses used the very same beds to comfort and treat patients. My informants spoke with pride about what seemed like ordinary household chores, an indication of how they valued their work at the same time as emphasising how their daily work was different from other women's jobs.

It was more than the above aspects of nursing associated with women's work that they highlighted. Nurses underscored how their daily work within colonial hospital settings elasticised and pushed the boundaries and meanings of nursing. Nurses entered nursing school with a simplified version of their responsibilities. To their surprise, their work also included aspects of medical work. Evidence shows that African women, just as the earlier generation of nursing orderlies, practised medical techniques and used medical technologies that in normal circumstances and at the time were a preserve for medical doctors, who were mostly men. At the same time, an examination of their work, especially beyond the gaze of the authorities, enables us to appreciate how women in clinical spaces played an important role in blurring the dichotomies between nursing and medical practices. As early as 1945, Sr Freeborn complained to the 1945 Health Commission of nursing assistants who were conducting laboratory work and could decide, 'whether a patient has malaria or bilharzia or anything else'.[88] The microscope was a gendered technology. It was mainly the preserve of men, especially doctors and the newly trained African microscopists. Nursing assistants had no formal training in using the microscope and in disease diagnosis. However, beyond the gaze of medical authorities, African nursing assistants turned themselves into 'medical authorities'. M. D. Moyo who worked at Bonda Mission Hospital in the 1950s remembered that part of her job description moved beyond merely the nursing of patients. She also played an important role in medical procedures at the rural clinic. She recalled giving 'anaesthetics and was surprised to get good results almost every time'.[89] Phaina Nyanhanda had this to say:

> We were trained for the situation in rural areas where doctors were hardly available. We were expected to be the main authority most of the times. Our training made sure that we could do many functions that if all things being normal, were supposed to be the realm of medical doctors. I for example, know how to take ex-rays and analyse them; take blood samples, giving anaesthesia, putting intravenous hydrotherapy. I am also well knowledgeable with suturing lacerations and my friends who worked at a TB unit were well competent in diagnosing TB through x-ray readings and sputum analysis. One would expect such clinical practices to be performed by specialists but at our nursing school, we were taught all these things in case we end up at hospitals or clinics where doctors only came once in a month. While the government did not pay us accordingly, we were superior in terms of our work as it went just beyond the daily ward experience.[90]

In most of my interviews, nurses emphasised how they encroached upon what seemed like medical work. While others specialised, for example, in surgical nursing, some of my informants suggested that they nevertheless managed to conduct work reserved for specialists.[91] Taking X-Rays, sputum tests and minor surgeries became new areas in which nurses practised their work. African nurses scrambled boundaries between medicine and nursing, at the same time gradually turning clinical spaces into their own. An emphasis on these activities by my informants points to the various ways in which concepts of nursing were being reshaped in the colonies. For example, in 1965, the national doctor-patient ratio for urban areas was 1:1,885 and the national average was 1:9,000.[92] The shortage of medical personnel, therefore, enabled African nurses to claim clinical spaces as their own, in the process encroaching upon work which was supposedly the preserve of medical authorities.

Bridging the cultural divide in clinical spaces

Hospitals were unique colonial institutions to many Africans. They were spaces for healing as much as they were spaces where people came to die. Their employees handled the most intimate body products and claimed great expertise through their knowledge and their use of medical technologies. For many nursing students, the introduction to the hospital culture began a journey that was to shape the rest of their lives. It was a point of no return; a route that was to distinguish them from traditional healers. Having access to clinical knowledge and being able to use clinical technologies to diagnose and treat patients, no doubt elevated nurses above indigenous healers. Within a short period of their arrival at the nursing school, young African women were introduced into the hospital culture. In most cases, as my informants indicated, they were not given enough time to be settled. It was business as usual for matrons who, according to Nyaradzo Buzengwe, were eager to weed out what they considered, 'unintelligent girls (young women) who had by chance found themselves in the programme'.[93] While it is not clear whether it was intentional on the part of the superiors to purge the programme of unfit students, the process itself left a profound impact on those who remained in nursing. It gave them an experience that helped in shaping their identity as nurses and created a bond amongst young African women who came from different parts of the country. The shared experience made nurses and nursing a prestigious profession, a profession that, as argued in the previous chapter, showed that African women were prepared to embrace changes within Rhodesian society whilst simultaneously pushing cultural boundaries in Rhodesia.

Nursing enabled African nurses to act as cultural brokers. As 'middles', to borrow from Nancy Rose Hunt, nurses used their position within clinical spaces to translate western medicine to Africans, whilst using their cultural understanding of disease causation and symptoms in translating African illnesses to their superiors. A central issue that affected nurses' work was related to disease diagnosis. Nurses I interviewed indicated that a significant proportion of patients they nursed during this time frequently failed to explain their ailments clearly. At times, African patients suppressed vital information. It was their responsibility to acquire the correct information for doctors and to make the diagnosis easier. Flora Matondo's response indicated that disease diagnosis and treatment within western hospitals was often complicated by the descriptions given of symptoms, and at times a different understanding of disease causation:

> Some patients were not clear in explaining what was affecting them, they might talk about – *chipotswa* – characterised by the sensation of an object moving rhythmically from one part of the body to another, for example from the left ear to the right groin. The periodicity may vary from one minute to a week and they usually say they experience painful sensations.[94]

It is evident that such descriptions of ailments were frustrating to most nurses. It presented them with a big challenge on the best way to treat patients.

Furthermore, failure to accurately describe ailments also presented a challenge in translating the information to their superiors, often white male doctors. The most common way of diagnosing unexplainable ailments in a western clinical setting would be to rely on lab results. However, in the 1950s and 1960s, not every patient in Rhodesia found their blood samples forwarded to the lab. In most cases, medical personnel relied on Africans' explanation of ailments. In clinical spaces, therefore, African nurses became the immediate vehicle for transferring such information. Flora Matondo and others maintained that if they suspected an ailment they were familiar with, they would suggest it to the doctor.[95] African nurses' presence within hospitals was reassuring for many patients that they were being nursed by their own. Towards this end, nurses drew upon their cultural understanding of disease causation in helping patients understand and negotiate different healthcare options.[96] Just as in other parts of the continent and like their predecessors, African nurses in Rhodesia thus played a pivotal role as cultural brokers between African and western health systems.[97] As interlocutors, nurses played a more critical role in shaping how the afflicted experienced colonial medicine, even though they enjoyed less authority and power than their European counterparts.

Working in hospitals meant that many nurses crossed their cultural nursing boundaries, in the process reshaping their understanding of taking care of the sick and helping the infirm. Nurses had to adjust to seeing, on a daily basis, strangers' bodies, especially male bodies, to probing healthy and diseased private parts as part of their work, and for some who took up surgical nursing as their speciality later in life, to continuously assist in the theatre and with surgical operations of different sorts. Nursing older patients presented a major cultural challenge to young African women. Historically, older women were the fulcrum of the care economy in rural areas. Young women, as noted in previous chapters, only acted in the role of helpers. The introduction of hospitals and the subsequent entrance of young women into clinical spaces partly transferred the care economy from the private sphere into the public domain. The presence of hospitals also shifted the burden of nursing from older women to younger women. When older women and men attended clinical spaces, they were now deferring to younger women.[98] Young women possessed western knowledge over diseases, the knowledge that partly drew African patients to hospitals. Furthermore, young women had access to hospital technologies to diagnose diseases. They wore uniforms that were a signifier of authority over disease diagnosis and remedies to be followed within hospitals. But, as many acknowledged, nursing older patients, especially strangers, brought a sense of anxiety on their part. Treating older patients in clinical spaces presented a cultural challenge these young nurses had to overcome. Tsitsi Chinamasa remembered that feeding and later giving shots was not a problem at all. However, her primary issue was being asked to bathe a patient who was as old as her father. She dutifully accomplished the task but said it made her feel uncomfortable the whole day.[99] Of course, with time, nurses got used to conducting these tasks without much anxiety. Thus, while young nurses were pushing the boundaries of traditional understandings of nursing through their presence in clinical spaces, the normalisation of their earlier anxieties can also be viewed as a way in which they were reshaping their cultural understandings of nursing.

Some patients made it difficult for young nurses to adjust to clinical practice. Information from interviews suggests that older patients were also uncomfortable with such arrangements. With the increased visits of males to hospitals, it became a question of the extent to which older men would be willing to allow younger women access to their sick bodies. Veronica Sibanda remembered how it was difficult for her in her first years of nursing to take care of elderly male patients: 'Unlike today you could see that they were reluctantly allowing you to take care of them. They acquiesce because they had no choice.'[100] While not many encountered patients who refused to be nursed, a letter in the *African Weekly* brings out what might have been a source of major tension between nurses and patients at Harari Hospital: the refusal to disclose information to younger nurses by the elderly. Written by a 'young man' the letter gave praise to young African female nurses for their sterling work at the hospital. At the same time, it questioned the behaviour of older men in their conduct towards young African nurses. It read in part:

> I was admitted at Harari Hospital this month and was put into one of the surgery wards where the behaviour of the female nurses was most complimentary. Although I personally do not mind the treatment by female nurses as a young man, I noticed that the ward was full of elderly men who expressed a resenting impression of being treated by young female nurses. In some cases, these old men were refusing treatment. In general discussion with these elderly patients, I was informed that these men were very unhappy to entrust their private complaints to female nurses. Regarding the young female nurses as their 'daughters', these old men expressed the feeling that according to old African etiquette, an elderly man would not confide the secret causes of his illness to a person of his 'daughter's' age. As I saw it, it seems as though these elderly were not receiving appropriate treatment as they may have been shy to tell the female nurses the real position of their illness. The old men also expressed the fear that these young girls (young women) are allowed to meddle with their bodies in a genuine attempt to apply the medical treatment, they nevertheless lose the respect of these elderly men who by custom they are expected to respect.[101]

Such incidents exposed the complexity of nurse–patient relationships in a period of cultural change. Nurse–patient relationships were not straightforward, but contingent upon varied factors such as age and gender. Older patients' behaviour at Harari Hospital, for example, enables us to appreciate patients' role in the healing process. Their acceptance/rejection of medicine had an impact on nurses' work. The client-nurse relationship was often based on conflict and struggle. In this case, it was both a cultural and generational struggle. As in the Congo, 'maternity clinics and hospitals were and remained sites of debates and negotiation, translation and mistranslation, men and women challenged and transfigured the healthcare they received through complex processes of struggle, bargaining and compromise'.[102] Likewise, such an observation could be applied to clinical spaces in Rhodesia.

Young African women dismantled other taboos to make themselves comfortable in clinical spaces. According to my informants, traditionally, young women who helped the elderly in nursing were expected to avoid touching blood.[103] In her recollections of her teenage days, Laiza Shumba suggested that 'in those days, young women had to avoid being in contact with blood to avoid *kurwara* (to be sick)'.[104] In this case, Laiza Shumba claimed that taboo was linked to women's fears of experiencing menstruation problems and probably with conceiving.[105] In addition, young women were expected to avoid being in contact with dead bodies.[106] Again, Laiza Shumba remarked:

> Unlike today, attending funerals was not allowed when we were growing up. It was only our parents who would go. We would only attend funerals after getting married because by then you will be a mature person and having more responsibilities. But today, even children attend funerals. That was unheard of during our teenage years[107]

Since most of my informants came from rural areas, the mortality rates during that time in relation to the population were probably lower than today. Funerals were fewer and far apart. Thus, a significant proportion of nurses I interviewed indicated that they had their first sight of dead bodies at the hospital, something that was a novel phenomenon for many. Hence, when she entered training school, Jane Mushando was shocked that they had to be involved in the operating theatre and the idea that part of the nursing curriculum involved a post-mortem.[108] Hospitals were spaces in which African women, either as workers and/or as patients, experienced significant cultural shifts.

Despite the glamour and prestige associated with nursing, the issue of handling dead bodies made most student nurses in training schools anxious and nervous. Phaina Nyanhanda spoke for many when she said,

> I had problems and it was terrifying for me. During those times, when a relative passed away, we would not go to funerals unless it was a very close relative. Thus, I had never seen a dead body myself, and this was the most frightening thing that happened to me.[109]

Equally, Jane Mushando said that the issues related to handling dead bodies caused some of her relatives to advise her against entering the profession. They preferred her to enter the teaching profession. According to Jane Mushando, her relatives said that it was not their custom:

> As young women we were not allowed to handle dead bodies, especially strangers. In my village children were not allowed to attend funerals until they were older, about 15 years onwards. Even when we attended funerals, we were side-lined during body viewing, unless of course it was our closest relatives. In my case, when I told them I wanted to join nursing; they were not enthusiastic and cited issues concerning dead bodies. I think the bone of the contention was centred on handling men's dead bodies.[110]

Jane Mushando had no idea why some of these taboos were still prevalent in the society; she only wanted to go into the nursing profession. Even when her family had converted to Christianity, Jane Mushando maintained that such taboos were respected.

> It was just part of our culture that you would not expect a young girl to handle dead bodies, especially males. To make matters worse, to handle strange dead people! Maybe they thought that we might be affected by their spirits or something like that. I am not sure but just speculating. You see, we have what is called *ngozi* (avenging spirits) in Shona. Maybe they thought that if we failed to do our job properly, like being negligent and someone dies, then we would experience *ngozi* in our family. Probably that is why my relatives tried to dissuade me from going to nursing school. However, I was adamant and said to myself, this is what I want so I will do that no matter what people want. They later on said that I had made a good choice.

Anxieties over the possibilities of handling dead bodies were common among many nurses. While M. D. Moyo, who entered nursing school in 1939, was elated with the prospect for her job especially the maternity cases, she was always bothered by fear, especially the possibility of being in contact with dead bodies. 'Though I liked my work, fear was a bother. The first operation I attended was an eye surgery. That did not frighten me so much. The worst thing I dreaded was a corpse. Sister treated me. How? Well, I was forced to sleep in the Chapel when there was a dead body. The next morning all my fear was gone.'[111] For many informants, access to strangers' bodies became a rite of passage that differentiated them from other workers.

M. D. Moyo did not mention anything to do with the dissection of cadavers as the rite of passage for nurses in the colony. This did not suggest the unavailability of facilities and necessary equipment to carry out dissections and post-mortems. Facilities for dissection were available and there were unclaimed bodies that could have been used in the instruction for nurses and orderlies. However, as in East Africa, it is possible that instructors preferred using models as a precaution against suspicions of cannibalism and sorcery.[112] In her work, *Speaking with vampires*, Luise White noted how a cultural language of vampire stories emerged in East Africa. These stories grew out of a set of beliefs and practices of witchcraft, and they were part and parcel of Africans' way of making meaning of a new medical system.[113] Parallel cases existed in Rhodesia. The case of Dr Gurney is illustrative of African suspicions of cannibalism on the part of medical staff, especially doctors who performed autopsies. Following the instructions of the Native Commissioner, Dr Gurney of Old Umtali Mission hospital performed several autopsies in cases of sudden and violent deaths. In trying to come to terms with such acts, rumour circulated amongst Africans that 'he was eating the vital organs of the corpses he had examined'.[114] Suspicions alienated a significant number of Africans from his care. Although this was an isolated event at one mission station, one can speculate that such reactions also took place at other mission stations across the country. There is also a possibility that during the training of nursing assistants in the pre-war period, hospital authorities at mission hospitals deliberately used dummies *in lieu* of cadavers to teach African nursing orderlies anatomy. Such a reading helps us to come to terms with the absence of lab and cadaver stories in older informants.

While this was the experience for the first generation of nursing orderlies, by the 1950s, with the quest for having what was termed an ideal nurse, a nurse who would be in charge of rural clinics, it became imperative for new nursing schools to introduce nursing students to central aspects of biomedicine. The first-hand experience of human anatomy was one of the requirements of biomedical training. The training of nurses was not merely in the art of caring and everyday ward management. One of the issues that came out of the 1945 National Health Services Commission was the urgent need to improve nursing education in the country. Nursing education had to move away from just concentrating on domestic duties in the profession. It also had to introduce more sophisticated aspects of nursing to young African women. Thus, while some authorities urged that nurses concentrate on hygiene and domestics, farsighted medical doctors began to argue for specialised nursing like surgical and neurological nursing.[115] To achieve this, a deeper understanding of human physiology and anatomy was necessary.[116]

When she entered the anatomy lab at her nursing school for the first time, Christina Banda remembered the colour of the room. Its whiteness matched her uniform and was representative of cleanliness. It was also a depiction of the innocence she associated with the profession. However, the same space of healing was also a space of death. It was within the anatomy labs that many nurses were also to experience the horror of death and these experiences were central in reshaping their cultural understanding of nursing and their new perceptions of nursing ingrained in their memories for a long time. Christina Banda vividly remembered her experience in the anatomy lab, an experience that at times traumatised and unsettled her and her colleagues:

> My biggest problem was when we had to go to the mortuary for a post mortem. The man had committed suicide and the very nature of his death scared me. It was just two weeks after we had started school and it was something that everyone had to do irrespective of whether you liked or not. It was easy I think for those who had seen dead bodies or those who once worked in the mortuary like my friend who had been a nursing orderly the previous two years. When they dissected the cadaver, it was one of the most horrible things I have ever seen. I do not know how I managed as I was terrified. I remember some of my colleagues fainted and it was always the case even in years to come that some young women would find it hard to get through their first experience of the post-mortem. After that, I thought of leaving nursing, but I was told that I would get used to [it]. I spent two years without eating meat and we would usually sleep with lights on, as we were scared that the person will come back for us.[117]

Phaina Nyanhanda had an almost identical story:

> My first experience of seeing a dead person was at the hospital. I will not forget it, his name was Yotamu. We were instructed to go to the post-mortem room where they were dissecting him. They were doing that whilst we were watching, being shown every body part, heart and other internal organs. They later dissected the brain, showing us what it looked like. I did not sleep that night. It was very difficult for me to sleep. At one time, I left

the room to vomit. It was shocking. That night I did not eat. I just looked at the meat in my plate and felt as if I was going to eat Yotamu's flesh. It is only *varoyi* (witches) who eat people's flesh and I thought by eating meat that day I would become *muroyi* (witch). I had problems with sleeping. During the night, I fell from my bed. All I could see was Yotamu coming to me. I almost left training. Two trainees left. I wanted to follow suit but what would I do in the rural areas. To herd cattle? No, I decided to stay. We later got used to that but it was difficult. People used to say that we were drugged so that we see (*kuona*) and assist in the operation, but it was not that, we only got used to it.[118]

Nurses drew upon their cultural repertoires to make sense of their new world. Phaina Nyanhanda's reference to *varoyi* (witches) and the reason for her disinclination to eat meat for some time, points to the way she was trying to come to terms with her new clinical experience. To contextualise, amongst the Shona, not only does witchcraft bring misfortune, but also a – *muroyi* (witch) is an agent of death. *Muroyi* brings grief and disharmony in the community hence the proverb – *muroyi, royera kure / ugowana anokuviga* (witch, bewitch far away / that you may find someone to bury you) was meant to remind a *muroyi* to live in peace with his/her neighbours. *Varoyi* are also associated with cannibalism. For Phaina Nyanhanda, Christina Banda and others who might have had similar experiences in the post-mortem lab, visceral experience of dissected cadavers shocked them. Student nurses tried to come to terms with this new experience by explaining it culturally. By claiming that she is not a *muroyi* (not that anyone accused her of being that) I argue, she found a way of distancing herself from such practices whilst simultaneously asserting the opposite of what the *varoyi* do. By not eating meat and making connections between Yotamu and witchcraft, she was affirming her new role as a healer and sustainer of life rather than an agent of death.

Nurses' first experiences in the post-mortem lab and cadaver stories punctuated the reminiscences of their student days. These cadaver experiences in various forms brought home the realities of death for many. The experiences also had some repercussions for nursing students, implications that separated them from traditional caregiving intricacies that created a boundary between traditional medical practitioners and these new practitioners, who were taking over from their grandmothers and mothers in the art of caregiving. It also exposed and revealed to students the intricacies of the human body in ways that traditional healing practitioners had not yet experienced. As Illife noted in the case of East Africa, the various forms of cadaver experiences also taught nursing students to separate objectivity from emotions.[119] These places of death, the anatomy lab and the mortuaries, became special places. Having access to these spaces on a regular basis made nursing staff special people. Just as the hospital work itself, access to these areas that were closed to the public and general staff, was important in separating nursing staff from the rest of the hospital staff. It also separated them from the rest of the population that did not have access to such spaces, in the process helping to foster a common sense of identity amongst the nursing staff and the prospective nursing staff. Cadaver experiences, therefore, represented a status change for nurses. As pointed out, they represented a threshold crossed, 'a symbolic rite of passage into the hallowed realm of medicine'.[120] Their first experience with dead bodies in the mortuary and working with morticians was always a challenge. However, such experiences no doubt separated them from other workers and in the process helped in the changing social values.

Conclusion

The gradual transformations within Rhodesian Nursing Services that took place in the post-Second World War period had significant implications for government hospitals. The period saw the Africanisation of hospital spaces, which came into full swing in the 1960s. What started with the formal training of nursing aides and midwives was followed by the sending out of young African women to be trained in South Africa together with the commencement of the training of coloureds and people of Asian descent in 1953 and Africans in 1958. As a result, the Africanisation saw non-European women becoming the spine of nursing services from the 1960s onwards. However, the Africanisation process was more than having additional Africans as formally trained nurses within government hospitals. It also entailed the appointment of some Africans into senior positions within nursing services, in the process allowing them an opportunity to demonstrate their expertise and providing African nurses with the hope of future possibilities.

Even so, hospital spaces during the time under discussion remained quintessentially colonial spaces. Thus, irrespective of the Africanisation process, colonial relations were maintained within hospitals, with white medical and nursing personnel wielding power over a host of the non-European workforce. The case of student nurses, who traded one form of patriarchal control with another, and their struggles for independence, is a testament to the continuation of colonial relations within hospitals. When they transitioned into fulltime nurses and with some of their colleagues being elevated to more senior positions, African women remained subordinate in the colonial hospital setting. Still, in their subordinate positions, African nurses claimed the hospital spaces as their own. Being on the frontline of caring, African nurses shouldered the burden of nursing the sick in Rhodesian clinical spaces.

Furthermore, African nurses played an essential role in translating biomedical practices to Africans in Rhodesia. At the same time, nursing provided a new space where women could cross the cultural divide. The handling of dead bodies and participation in surgical operations and their presence in autopsy rooms was, for most of the informants, a novel phenomenon. To them, it was a demonstration of their entrance into the hallowed world of nursing. It was a testimony, a marker of difference between the new healing system anchored in biomedical practices and colonial hospitals, and the traditional understanding about bodies, blood and the entire healing process. References to the fear of touching corpses or being next to the medical doctor at the operating table indicated how the African nurse was encountering novel healing methods and also gives a reflection of the changing ideas of nursing amongst Africans in Rhodesia. The experiences of the 1960s generation set the tenor of the expected hospital work within African hospitals. It set precedents in terms of expectations – from patients and their relatives. While expectations were set, Rhodesian hospitals and nursing were to encounter numerous problems as a result of the political challenges the nation faced in the 1970s. The challenges had a significant impact on the practice of nursing within hospitals.

Notes

1. Gelfand, *A service to the sick*, p. 151.
2. For other countries see, for example H. Bell, 'Midwifery training and female circumcision in the inter war Anglo-Egyptian Sudan', *Journal of African History*, 39: 2 (1998), pp. 293–312; Vaughan, *Curing their ills* and Hunt, *A colonial lexicon*.
3. Interview: Mrs Laiza Shumba, Mabelreign Harare, 26 October 2008.
4. Gelfand, *A service to the sick*, p. 152.
5. See Masakure, 'One of the most serious problems'.
6. NAZ F 242/SM/300/20, Nursing during the Federal Era. A. O'Connor on behalf of the Medical Director, Letter to the Medical Superintendent Bulawayo Central Hospital, 'Training of Coloured and Asiatic Students at Bulawayo Central Hospital', 3 February 1960.
7. It is important to note that when Harari and Impilo were opened, white nursing students took some of their classes at these nursing schools as some of the best qualified tutors moved to African hospitals. Even when they took some of their classes at these schools, separation of races remained outside clinical spaces.
8. NAZ Annual Report on the Public Health which covers Northern Rhodesia, Nyasaland and Southern Rhodesia, (1954).
9. NAZ F 242/SM/300/20, Nursing during the Federal Era. L. P. Harrington, Medical Superintendent, Bulawayo Central Hospital, Letter to the Director of Medical Services, 'Training of Coloured and Asiatic Students at Bulawayo Central Hospital', 13 July 1960.
10. NAZ F 242/SM/300/20, Nursing during the Federal Era. L. P. Harrington, Medical Superintendent Bulawayo Central Hospital, Letter to the Director of Medical Services, 'Training of Coloured and Asiatic Students at Bulawayo Central Hospital', 13 July 1960.
11. NAZ F 242/SM/300/20, Nursing during the Federal Era. A. O'Connor on behalf of the Medical Director, Letter to the Medical Superintendent Bulawayo Central Hospital, 'Training of Coloured and Asiatic Students at Bulawayo Central Hospital', 3 February 1960.
12. NAZ F 242/SM/300/20, Nursing during the Federal Era. A. O'Connor on behalf of the Medical Director, Letter to the Medical Superintendent Bulawayo Central Hospital, 'Training of Coloured and Asiatic Students at Bulawayo Central Hospital', 3 February 1960.
13. By the end of the war, the government had approved plans to build two major African referral hospitals in Bulawayo and Salisbury. The Bulawayo, to be named Mpilo (life) was going to cater for the southern half of the country, and Harari Central Hospital for northern provinces. At the same time, the government began expanding district hospitals in Umtali and Gwelo with the anticipation that in future they would be central hospitals

and therefore have the capacity to house more patients and be advanced enough to train SRNs.
14 Gelfand, *A service to the sick*, p. 149.
15 For more on the politics of the Federation see, C. Leys and C. Pratt (eds), *A new deal in Central Africa* (London: Heinemann, 1960).
16 Leys and Pratt (eds), *A new deal in Central Africa*.
17 B. Chidzero, 'The meaning of good government in Central Africa', in C. Leys and C. Pratt (eds), *A new deal in Central Africa*, pp. 170–80.
18 C. Leys, '"Partnership" as the dismantling of colour bar', Leys and Pratt (eds), *A new deal in Central Africa*, pp. 98–109.
19 Interview: Mrs Laiza Shumba, Mabelreign Harare, 26 October 2008; Mrs Flora Matondo, Sakubva Mutare, 12 August 2008.
20 Interviews: Mrs Laiza Shumba, Mabelreign Harare, 26 October 2008; Mrs Flora Matondo, Sakubva Mutare, 12 August 2008.
21 NAZ SM/300/Ingut- Ingutsheni Hospital Nursing Staff: General.
22 Interviews: Mrs Laiza Shumba, Mabelreign Harare, 26 October 2008; Mrs Flora Matondo, Sakubva Mutare, 12 August 2008.
23 Interview: Mrs Flora Matondo, Sakubva Mutare, 12 August 2008.
24 Interview: Mrs Flora Matondo, Sakubva Mutare, 12 August 2008.
25 Interview: Mrs Flora Matondo, Sakubva Mutare, 12 August 2008.
26 *The African Weekly*, 4 January 1961.
27 *The African Weekly*, 25 January 1961.
28 Interviews: Mrs Laiza Shumba, Mabelreign Harare, 26 October 2008; Ms Esther Mawoyo, Chikanga Mutare, 22 February 2009; Mrs Nyaradzo Buzengwe, Harare, 10 July 2009.
29 *Central African Journal of Medicine*, 'Promotion of the first African State Registered Nurses to the grade of sister in the Federal Government Nursing Service', 8: 7 (1962), pp. 279–80.
30 *Central African Journal of Medicine*, 'Promotion of the first African State Registered Nurses to the grade of sister in the Federal Government Nursing Service', 8: 7 (1962), pp. 279–80.
31 *Central African Journal of Medicine*, 8: 10 (1962), p. 400.
32 S. Nzenza, *Zimbabwean woman: My own story* (London: Karia Press, 1988), pp. 67–9.
33 The contracts student nurses signed when entering nursing school described them as minors, who, when in signing the contract, were expected to have been 'duly assisted by her Parent and Guardian...', See NAZ F 122/FH/190/51, Government of the Federation of Rhodesia and Nyasaland, Ministry of Health, Branch 1, Contract: Student Nurses.
34 Schmidt, *Peasants, traders and wives*.
35 Interviews: Mrs Laiza Shumba, Chikanga Mutare, 22 February 2009; Ms Esther Mawoyo, Mabelreign Harare, 26 October 2008; Mrs Nyaradzo Buzengwe, Harare, 10 July 2009. This was a running theme that came out of the interviews and it cut across generations.

36 Interviews: Mrs Laiza Shumba, Chikanga Mutare, 22 February 2009; Ms Esther Mawoyo, Mabelreign Harare, 26 October 2008; Mrs Nyaradzo Buzengwe, Harare, 10 July 2009.
37 Nzenza, *Zimbabwean woman*, p. 67.
38 Nzenza, *Zimbabwean woman*, pp. 68–9.
39 Melosh, *The physician's hand*, p. 37.
40 Interview: Mbuya Phaina Nyanhanda, Harare, 15 August 2007. Interview by P. Mukwambo.
41 Interview: Mrs Laiza Shumba, Mabelreign Harare, 26 October 2008.
42 A comparison of the rules today and at the time when Mrs Laiza Shumba trained as a nurse reveals differences in rules. Unlike in the past where aspiring nursing students had to submit reference letters from their teachers on their 'moral character', later aspiring nursing students had to submit their grades only. Furthermore, while some nursing students stay on campus, the majority of present-day nursing students stay out of campus.
43 *The African Weekly*, 4 January 1961.
44 *The African Weekly*, 5 July 1961.
45 Robert Mugabe, who had a driver's licence, drove Msipa back home. C. G. Msipa, *In pursuit of freedom and justice: A memoir* (Harare: Weaver Press, 2015), pp. 30–1.
46 *The African Weekly*, 4 January 1961.
47 *The African Weekly*, 12 July 1961.
48 Nzenza, *Zimbabwean woman*, pp. 67–9. Even in independent Zimbabwe, such policy continued for some time. For example in his one-year reign as the Minister of Health in independent Zimbabwe, H. Ushewokunze dismissed a total of forty-five unmarried nursing students from the service. G. W. Sedman, 'Women in Zimbabwe: Post independence struggles', *Feminist Studies*, 10: 3 (1984), pp. 419–40.
49 Interview: Mrs Flora Matondo, Sakubva Mutare, 12 August 2008.
50 Interview: Mrs Flora Matondo, Sakubva Mutare, 12 August 2008.
51 L. J. Ross, 'African-American women and abortion: A neglected history', *Journal of Health Care for the Poor and Underserved*, 3: 2 (1992), pp. 274–84.
52 A. Kaler, *Running after their pills: Politics, gender and contraception in colonial Zimbabwe* (Portsmouth, NH: Heinemann, 2003), pp. 48–9.
53 Kaler, *Running after their pills*, p. 61.
54 Interview: Mrs Nelia Ncube, Chitungwiza, 20 April 2009.
55 For more see Kaler, *Running after their pills*.
56 Interview: Mrs Laiza Shumba, Mabelreign Harare, 26 October 2008.
57 Interview: Mrs Laiza Shumba, Mabelreign Harare, 26 October 2008.
58 Interview: Mrs Laiza Shumba, Mabelreign Harare, 26 October 2008.
59 NAZ F 242/SM/300/20, Nursing during the Federation, 'Training of Student Nurses'.

60 NAZ F 242/SM/300/20, Nursing during the Federation, 'Schedule of Training: Impilo and Harari'.
61 NAZ F 242/SM/300/20, Nursing during the Federation, 'Schedule of Training: Impilo and Harari'.
62 Interviews: Mrs Flora Matondo, Sakubva Mutare 12 August 2008; Mrs Veronica Sibanda, Harare, 15 September 2008; Mrs Fadzai Mugove, Harare 10 July 2008. Over the course of forty-eight months, their day duty was organised as follows: three months each: children's surgical ward, female or male ward, orthopaedic ward, general ward – male or female, children's medical ward, male specialist ward, genital urinary ward and operating theatre. Two months were spent in the outpatient and casualty ward. Night duty was organised as follows: three months at a time, twelve nights on and three off. The night-duty work was, for example: first year as a junior in children's medical or surgical ward, second year as a junior in female or male medical ward, third year in charge of gynaecological ward under supervision of the night superintendent, fourth year in charge of male surgical ward under the supervision of the night superintendent.
63 NAZ LG 191/12/7/88. Ante Natal Care; Illegal residents, Harari Township. Council Minutes 9 March 1954. For more see for example, Barnes, 'We women worked so hard'.
64 For more see Barnes, 'We women worked so hard'.
65 NAZ LG 191/12/7/88, Ante natal care: Illegal residents, Harari Township. Council Minutes 9 March 1954.
66 NAZ LG 191/12/7/88, Letter from J. M. Blair, Director of Medical Services dated 23 August 1954 to the Town Clerk. Ref: Ante natal care: Illegal residents: Harari Township.
67 H. S. Gear, 'Some problems of the medical services of the Federation of Rhodesia and Nyasaland', *British Medical Journal*, 2 (1960), pp. 525–31.
68 Interview: Mrs Laiza Shumba, Mabelreign Harare, 26 October 2008.
69 Interview: Ms Esther Mawoyo, Chikanga Mutare, 22 February 2009.
70 All of my informants emphasised this.
71 Interview: Mrs Jane Mushando, Sakubva Mutare, 27 April 2009.
72 Interview: Mrs Jane Mushando, Sakubva Mutare, 27 April 2009.
73 Interview: Mrs Jane Mushando, Sakubva Mutare, 27 April 2009.
74 NAZ F 242/SM/300/20, Nursing during the Federation, 'Schedule of Training: Impilo and Harare Hospitals'.
75 Interview: Mrs Flora Matondo, Sakubva Mutare, 12 August 2008.
76 See for example, Munyaradzi and Muronda, 'Some attitudes of patients discharged from Harare Hospital', and Kavumbura and Mossop, 'Attitudes to illness in Salisbury, 1980'.
77 J. Janzen, *The quest for therapy: Medical pluralism in lower Zaire* (Berkeley: University of California Press, 1978), p. 4.

78 Jackson, *Surfacing up*, pp. 163–66.
79 Kavumbura and Mossop, 'Attitudes to illness in Salisbury', pp. 111–14.
80 Interviews: Mrs Flora Matondo, Sakubva Mutare, 12 August 2008 and Mrs Fadzai Mugove, Harare, 10 July 2008.
81 Interview: Mrs Veronica Sibanda, Harare, 15 September 2008.
82 Interview: Mrs Fadzai Mugove, Harare, 10 July 2008.
83 Interview: Mrs Fadzai Mugove, Harare, 10 July 2008.
84 Interview: Mrs Nyaradzo Buzengwe, Harare, 10 July 2009.
85 Interview: Mrs Nyaradzo Buzengwe, Harare, 10 July 2009.
86 Interviews: Mrs Nyaradzo Buzengwe, Harare, 10 July 2009; Ms Tsitsi Chinamasa, Old Mutare, 28 May 2009.
87 M. Sandelowski, *Devices and desires: Gender, technology, and American nursing* (Chapel Hill and London: The University of North Carolina Press, 2000), p. 45.
88 NAZ ZBP 2/1/4, National Health Services Commission. Sister L. Freeborn, Representing South African Nursing Association, Mashonaland Branch to the National Health Services Commission.
89 Letter from M. D. Moyo, Bonda Mission to M. Gelfand, undated, quoted in *A service to the sick*, p. 136.
90 Interview: Mbuya Phaina Nyanhanda, 15 August 2007. Interview by P. Mukwambo.
91 Interview: Mrs Dhlamini, Harare, 22 August 2008.
92 W. Fraser Ross, 'Nursing in Rhodesia, past, present and future' *Rhodesia Nurse* (1967), p. 32.
93 Interview: Mrs Nyaradzo Buzengwe, Harare, 10 July 2009.
94 Interview: Mrs Flora Matondo, Sakubva Mutare, 12 August 2009.
95 Interview: Mrs Flora Matondo, Sakubva Mutare, 12 August 2009.
96 Interviews: Mrs Flora Matondo, Sakubva Mutare, 12 August 2009; Mrs Nyaradzo Buzengwe, Harare, 10 July 2009; Mrs Laiza Shumba, Mabelreign Harare, 26 October 2008.
97 Digby and Sweet, 'Nurses as cultural brokers', pp. 113–29.
98 Interviews: Mrs Flora Matondo, Sakubva Mutare, 12 August 2009; Mrs Nyaradzo Buzengwe, Harare, 10 July 2009; Mrs Laiza Shumba, Mabelreign Harare, 26 October 2008.
99 Interview: Ms Tsitsi Chinamasa, Old Mutare, 28 May 2009.
100 Interview: Mrs Veronica Sibanda, Harare, 15 September 2008.
101 *The African Weekly*, 28 June 1961.
102 Hunt, *A colonial lexicon*, p. 8.
103 Interview: Mrs Laiza Shumba, Mabelreign Harare, 26 October 2008.
104 Interview: Mrs Laiza Shumba, Mabelreign Harare, 26 October 2008.
105 Interview: Mrs Laiza Shumba, Mabelreign Harare, 26 October 2008.
106 Interview: Mrs Laiza Shumba, Mabelreign Harare, 26 October 2008.

107 Interview: Mrs Laiza Shumba, Mabelreign Harare, 26 October 2008.
108 Interview: Mrs Jane Mushando, Sakubva Mutare, 27 April 2009.
109 Interview: Mbuya Phaina Nyanhanda, Harare, 15 August 2007.
110 Interview: Mrs Jane Mushando, Sakubva Mutare, 27 April 2009. Interview by P. Mukwambo.
111 Letter from M. D. Moyo, Bonda Mission to Michael Gelfand, undated, quoted in, *A service to the sick*, p. 136.
112 Illife, *East African doctors*, p. 74.
113 L. White, *Speaking with vampires: Rumor and history in Colonial Africa* (Berkeley: University of California Press, 2000). See Chapter 3: ' "Bandages on your mouth": The experience of colonial medicine in East and Central Africa'.
114 G. Downie, 'Methodist Hospital, Nyadiri (Washburn Memorial) past and present', *Central African Journal of Medicine*, 8: 2 (1960), pp. 69–71.
115 NAZ ZBP 1/2/4 National Health Services Commission, Miss Munro, Matron. Lady Chancellor Nursing Home. Oral evidence to the Commission dated 19 September 1945.
116 NAZ ZBP 1/2/4 National Health Services Commission, Miss Munro, Matron. Lady Chancellor Nursing Home. Oral evidence to the Commission dated 19 September 1945.
117 Interview: Mrs Christina Banda, Norton July 2009.
118 Interview: Mbuya Phaina Nyanhanda Harare, 15 August 2007. Interview by P. Mukwambo.
119 Illife, *The East African doctors*, p. 74.
120 J. W. Lela and D. Pawluch, 'Medical students and the cadaver in social and cultural context', in M. Lock and D. Gordon (eds), *Biomedicine examined* (London: Kluver Academic Publishers, 1988), pp. 125–53.

5

Nursing a nation at war: Nurses' experiences during the 1970s

Introduction

One of the central features of the 1970s decade was the liberation war, which started in earnest in 1972 and culminated with the Lancaster House Conference of 1979 that led to majority rule and independence in 1980. The war pitted the mainly white dominated Rhodesian government and the black dominated nationalists against each other. The war that resulted from the struggle between the nationalists and the minority government had a significant effect not only on race relations in Rhodesia. Thus, taking hospitals as a microcosm of the society, one notes that the challenges that faced the nation were also reflected within clinical spaces. During the 1970s, hospitals became sites of struggles fought in the political arena. The racial conflicts in hospitals during the 1970s reflected the tensions and anxieties that gripped a nation at war. To be specific, the government insisted on maintaining the policy informed by the strongest racial prejudice that limited the presence of Africans in wards at a time when it was becoming clear that they were failing to train enough personnel for white patients. While some members of the white community were adamant about the need for the policy to be maintained, some liberals within the white community and African legislators argued otherwise – exposing the contradictions within the policy and the impact of the policy on service provision. They called on the government to dismantle the policy and employ African nurses in white wards and hospitals. It was not until the second half of the decade that various government hospitals began employing African nurses for white wards. Such changes were in part a response to the government's failure to train enough white nurses, but also due to nursing staff attrition as a result of the war and the need on the part of the government to appease internal black nationalists.

The war had a direct impact on the provision of health services in hospitals. A significant number of white professionals left the country for various reasons, including security problems and to avoid the military draft. The exodus of white personnel further entrenched the Africanisation of clinical spaces that began in the 1950s. Furthermore, the war affected urban and rural hospitals in other ways. Urban hospitals experienced a surge in patients while rural hospitals came under immense pressure from warring parties. The war had a significant effect on the everyday work experiences of African nurses in hospitals. Rural nurses, on one hand, received threats from Rhodesian Security Forces and were at times arrested, tortured and beaten up for various reasons, including being suspected of aiding guerrillas, failure to report the presence of guerrillas, or failure to report suspected war casualties. On the other hand, guerrillas expected nurses to contribute in medicine or through other ways such as providing clothes. Nurses, just as peasants, juggled between two warring armies. In their recollections of the 1970s, African nurses stressed that their presence within clinical spaces was central in nursing a nation at war. By not abandoning their practice, rural nurses implicitly contributed to the liberation of the country. The inclusion of nurses within liberation struggle narratives is essential. The current historiography of the liberation struggle emphasises the nature of the struggle, with an examination of combatants, the war and its impact on peasant livelihoods. Often silenced in the literature was the impact of the liberation struggle on healthcare in Rhodesia.

Besides stoking racial tensions and transforming both urban and rural hospitals, the war also introduced new types of patients – casualties of war battles. The last wars fought on Rhodesian soil took place in 1893 and 1896, in the early years of colonial rule. The hospital system was still in its infancy. Thus until the 1970s, no war had been fought on Rhodesian soil. Except for the specialised military nurses, the majority of African nurses had never encountered war casualties. With time, black and white nursing staff 'became very efficient and adept at treating casualties and gunshot wounds'.[1] Besides bringing new challenges – nursing war casualties, the war introduced another health centre – the 'bush hospital'. The 'bush hospital' catered for the health needs of nationalist combatants and refugees in neighbouring countries. A number of the workers who provided medical and nursing services in the 'bush hospitals' had little experience in hospital work. Recruited from those Zimbabweans who had crossed the border to join the liberation forces, the majority of these hospital workers – nurses and medics – were in-house trained. With their limited training, these women and men creatively adapted to the war situation to provide medical services to their colleagues.

Racism in government hospitals in the 1970s

The struggles between Africans and Europeans have always been a central motif in Rhodesian history. Rhodesian society was built and sustained on the separation of races and a battery of legislation was enacted to control the contact between races. Efforts to limit racial contacts also extended to clinical spaces with hospital wards racially segregated. Furthermore, as noted in previous chapters, the Africanisation of the nursing profession in Rhodesia was partly based on the desire to maintain racial segregation. Specifically, it hinged on the need to limit white nurses' association with African patients. With an increased number of patients attending government hospitals, it became imperative that African nurses be trained to serve their people. As much as white nurses could tend to African patients, African nurses, however, were not expected to nurse white patients. It was the responsibility of white nurses, and at times, Asian and coloured nurses, to take care of white patients. This canon worked well with the availability of enough white, Asian or coloured nurses to tend to white patients. However, Rhodesia never produced enough nurses for this rule to work effectively.

The 1970s brought significant changes that put this rule to the test. In what had become the norm, hospital authorities were anxious about their failure to train enough personnel to tend to the white patients.[2] In addition, they were troubled by the enduring problem of the failure to retain trained white nurses. In her report to the Secretary for Health, the Matron of the United Bulawayo Hospitals praised the sterling work that her hospital was doing in producing brilliant students who have 'excelled themselves in the Republic of South Africa: Two having been awarded gold medals and three achieving passes with honours on completion of midwifery training.'[3] While she congratulated the nursing school for the high standards of nurses trained, she was quick to point out the perennial problem of nurses leaving for greener pastures and at times, resigning from service: 'It must be a cause of dissatisfaction, however, that such excellent nurses have decided to seek their midwifery training outside the country. Here again it is, unfortunately, necessary for me to record the large wastage of student nurses, and during the year 24 student nurses resigned before completing their contracts.'[4] Within such an environment of the continuous shortage of white nurses, the government maintained the policy that 'only European, coloured and Asian nurses may nurse European patients in government hospitals'[5] and only in emergency wards 'would African nurses be allowed to nurse European patients'.[6] This no doubt affected the provision of services to patients in government hospitals. For example, Rhodesians of European origin in Bindura, a farming town north-west of Salisbury, were outraged with government's failure to furnish the hospital with enough nurses to tend to white patients at the hospital.[7] As with other Rhodesian hospitals, Bindura Hospital was divided into two – the European and African sections. By the end of 1974, the fourteen-bed European section of the hospital was functioning with three nurses instead of seven.[8] The shortage of nurses (four white/coloured or Asian) had restricted the hospital services to the white community of the town to emergency cases and outpatient services only.[9] While the government managed to cover the gap by posting one African nurse to work in the African section of the hospital and three European nurses for the European section,[10] it was not only Bindura that was facing such a dire situation. Across the country, there were reports of some wards being closed. This was not because of the shortage of white patients, but due to the unavailability of nursing personnel deemed suitable to nurse white patients.[11] The scaling down of services to the white community of Bindura and the possibility of such a scenario being repeated in small town hospitals across the country reignited the debates over the need for the government to change its policy towards the nursing profession in the country. The problem at Bindura was not the unavailability of nurses. What was in short supply were European/Asian or coloured nurses who were allowed by policy to work in the white section of government hospitals.

It is important to appreciate that not all whites supported segregationist policies. In a sea of conservatism, liberals fought hard for their voice to be heard. One of those to attack this policy was Laurence Fraser Levy, Professor of Surgery at the University of Rhodesia. As early as 1962, Levy wrote a letter to *The Central African Journal of Medicine* celebrating the Federal Supreme Court's decision that struck down the segregation of swimming pools in the Federation. Levy urged the 'spring tide of desegregation' to be extended to clinical spaces.[12] Fifteen years down the line, Levy still maintained his stance, making a strong criticism of government's segregationist policies in clinical spaces. In his strongly worded letter to *The Rhodesia Herald* newspaper, Levy argued for an urgent policy shift and for progressive Rhodesians to embrace multiracialism in Rhodesian hospitals and outside clinical spaces. Levy wrote:

> It has been Government policy for many years that only European or Asian nurses shall nurse European patients in Government hospitals. Yet until recently, and I suspect still present, there have been more well trained African nurses; fully State Registered Nurses of the highest quality turned out by the schools at Harari and Impilo Central Hospitals than there were jobs for them. I have seen many of these desperate for work, and if the same situation does not still prevail, I shall be surprised. Even if it does not still prevail, the problems of staffing Bindura and other hospitals could be met in the longer run by increasing the number of African girls in training and employing them after qualification. There are many more suitable applicants for training than there are places available in the nursing school, whereas, it has been harder to persuade European girls to take up the profession.[13]

Unavailability of qualified nurses to work in white wards was not the main issue here. The crux of the matter was the unattainability of qualified nurses of certain races expected to work in white wards. The whole 'quality of African nurses' argument that was a thin veil in justifying clinical apartheid made no sense. Pointed out above by Levy, African nurses were equally qualified as white nurses or Asian nurses. For African nurses, therefore, their race was the cardinal sin that denied them the opportunity to tend to white patients.

The situation at Bindura and probably at other government hospitals across the country, was an entirely artificial one borne out of the strongest racial prejudice and policy. In 1975, the government reported that the all-white hospital, Andrew Fleming Hospital (AFH), had vacancies for fifty-one nurses. The Ministry of Health was failing to fill the posts.[14] In the same year, 1975, the government began constructing the second phase of the hospital. The government expected to complete constructing AFH in 1981.[15] At a time when African patients at Harari Hospital were crammed in wards with some sleeping on the floor and others being discharged early due to lack of accommodation, the conditions at AFH at its opening in 1973 were luxurious. Hospital wards had an average of four beds per room and the hospital had rooms 'designed to give flexibility as regards to sex of patients and specialty.'[16] However, considering government policy, the major challenge was staffing this luxurious hospital with the right kind of nurses. Already short of white nurses, vacancies at AFH had to be opened to every trained nurse regardless of race. Thus, there was every need on the part of authorities in particular and some members of the white community in general, to cease being narrow-minded and shift their attitude towards appreciating multiracialism and equality.

Multiculturalism entailed introducing a sea change in racial attitudes in every aspect of daily life. It was, therefore, hypocritical on the part of many who were unwilling to be nursed by African nurses yet on daily basis were in contact with Africans in the most intimate spaces: their homes. A history of domestic service in Rhodesia brings out this point very well. Domestic service was an important pillar of Rhodesian society. White homes were spaces where Africans had closer contact with Europeans. Flora Matondo suggested that she found it contradictory that 'the same white people were willing to eat food prepared by African hands and did not mind African nannies looking after their children. Yet they tried by all means to limit African nurses' presence in white hospitals.'[17] Just like Flora Matondo, progressives like Levy also pointed out such contradictions within Rhodesian society:

> Virtually every European family in this country live in close relationship with African servants of lower educational levels than these girls (nurses). How absurd is it not to be nursed by one of them when they are sick. The consequence of this bigoted and discriminatory policy is that both sides suffer. African girls cannot get jobs for which they have been trained and

some of the good people (white people) of Bindura cannot use their own hospital.[18]

There is no doubt that the policy compromised the provision of health services. However, some sections of the white community were averse to change and unwilling to shift their stance. Within two days of Levy's scathing attack of government policy and attitude, the Minister of Information defended the policy maintaining that only European and Asian nurses should nurse European patients in government hospitals.[19] Probably fearing to antagonise and upset the remaining white population that was central to the political survival of Ian Smith's government, the minister maintained that policy in government hospitals was not going to be eradicated.

One would have expected this policy to be followed in most clinical spaces in Rhodesia. However, it was not the case. Sometimes rules were ignored. A brief examination of the private sector exposes policy contradictions and the hypocrisy of some of the authorities bent on maintaining racial separation in government hospitals. By the early 1970s, the private sector had all but scrambled the policy devotedly followed in government hospitals. For example, African medical personnel diagnosed and treated white patients just as they did to African patients during the 1970s.[20] Dr Mzengezi's case immediately comes to mind. Dr Mzengezi practised medicine in Gwelo, the third biggest city. In 1972, the Minister of Local Government and Housing instructed Gwelo Town Council to furnish Mzengezi with a land tenure permit to set up his surgery in a designated white area under the 1934 Land Apportionment Act (revised in 1941). The Act decreed that, 'No Native (African) shall acquire, lease or occupy land in the European area.'[21] However, the government could make special cases, hence the Minister's request. Two years later, in 1974, the Gwelo City Council rescinded this decision. Mzengezi had to leave his premises and move to a designated African area; the Gwelo City Council reasoned that not only was Mzengezi's surgery in the wrong part of the town, but the presence of the surgery was attracting a large number of blacks to a white neighbourhood.[22] In his plea to maintain his surgery at the premises, Dr Mzengezi maintained that not only did he offer services to African patients, but that he also served members of the white community. He was allowed to stay at the premises and continued treating patients from all racial groups.[23] Mzengezi's case is important for it confirms that such racial boundaries in medical and nursing practices were at times scrambled even though some authorities were eager to prop them up. Here was an African medical doctor who served a multiracial society. Justifiably, he was a qualified doctor and patients, regardless of their race, trusted his services. It is also possible that his services were cheaper as compared to other medical doctors in the city. Of particular importance for this analysis is that Mzengezi employed African nurses as part of his staff.[24] These were the same nurses that officials and legislators restricted from nursing white patients in government hospitals. Just as happened in South Africa during the 1970s, private medical facilities in Rhodesia were at the forefront of eroding racial barriers within medical and nursing practice.[25] In South Africa, as in Rhodesia, the fulcrum of private hospitals, nursing homes and surgeries in the 1970s shifted from being mainly white, to employing coloureds and blacks. Even Levy acknowledged in his criticism of the policy that in Rhodesia, 'African girls have been doing so (nursing white patients) successfully for some years in private nursing homes'.[26]

The issue revolving around restricting African women from white wards was also raised in the Rhodesian parliament as African legislators added their voice for reforms. R. T. D. Sadomba was clear when he noted that a sizable proportion of the white community, including some ministers and legislators 'can go into some private hospitals who [sic] have decided to employ non-whites, and they have received good treatment'.[27] Sadomba saw it as a travesty of justice that:

> It should be Government policy that they cannot employ African nurses in white hospitals and wards. After all, there are some whites who have gone to be treated in the so called African hospitals if certain facilities were not available in European hospitals.[28]

African legislators in parliament were unanimous in their calls for the government to dismantle the policy. They maintained that African nurses be allowed to nurse white patients and above all, get equal treatment in promotions and other matters related to the profession.

The shortage of white nurses compelled private practitioners and private nursing homes to employ African nurses. Furthermore, it was cheaper for private practitioners and nursing homes to engage

African nurses as they would not be compelled to match the employment packages offered to white nurses in government hospitals.[29] Nelia Ncube remembered that African nurses who worked in private nursing homes earned higher wages in comparison to those working in government hospitals. Nevertheless, African nurses were still paid lower salaries in comparison to white nurses.[30] Interesting to note is that private hospitals conveniently disregarded the racial policy. Also, white patients who attended private doctors or hospitals were less bothered about who nursed them. It was government hospitals, the bastion of clinical apartheid that needed urgent reforms if hospitals were to continue providing quality care to patients. Yet authorities were unwilling to change the policy as they maintained that African nurses could not tend to white patients. Speaking on behalf of the white community, white MPs in the Rhodesian parliament were totally against the integration of hospital services and the idea that African nurses could nurse white patients. One of the legislators, Dr Barlow, felt that changing policy within hospitals would destroy the hallmark of the Rhodesian system. Barlow was not prepared to accept policy changes considering:

> The tremendous amount of work this Government has done to Africanise this service with African hospitals. And then one considers the discrimination and intimidation that takes place within these hospitals (African hospitals) by senior African staff against more junior European nurses, the Government is entirely right in its policy of providing European nurses in European hospitals and African nurses in African hospitals.[31]

With racism entrenched within Rhodesian society, it is not surprising that in the 1970s, a significant number still felt the need to preserve the racial divide in hospitals, especially between patients and nurses. Even though they were experiencing problems with the understaffing, they still held in reverence the place of the white nurse within clinical spaces and strongly felt that hospital integration would push white nurses from the nursing service.

Even though sections of the white population held tenaciously to segregationist ideas, it was becoming clear to Rhodesians by 1976 that change was imminent. Chiredzi Hospital is a good example of how hospital administrators took a two-pronged approach to deal with the shortage of white nurses for the white section of the hospital. First, they turned to white volunteers via the Red Cross to help with the day to day running of the hospital. The Provincial Medical Officer of Health of Victoria Province, indicated that besides white volunteers manning telephones, sitting with blood donors, organising refreshments when required, a group of Red Cross ladies:

> Has been attending lectures once a week. They have learnt the layout of the hospital, been taught how to make beds, give bed baths, take temperature, pulses and blood pressures and chart them. A brief lecture in Anatomy has helped them to identify the part of the body to be X-rayed when they have to escort patients to the X-ray department. They become very useful members of the Casevac teams and often assist in the European Hospital when it is very busy … This has relieved nursing staff to perform the more specialized work.[32]

Besides turning to non-professionals to assist with hospital work, it was the second approach that was an indicator of the changes that were to take place within hospitals. At Chiredzi, probably with the green light from medical officers, the hospital administrators turned to African nurses to nurse white patients. Again, the Provincial Medical Officer of Victoria Province, reported:

> The situation with nursing staff was difficult and the greatest problem was to find staff to cover the hospital (the white section of the hospital) on night duty. An eight-hour shift was started and a 40-hour week using African sisters to cover both hospitals (white and African) at night. This immediately improved the running of the hospital, and the staff settled into a happy working relationship and the public responded very well to the change.[33]

In September 1977, the Matabeleland Committee of the Rhodesia Medical Association pressed the government to implement policy changes arguing that 'there must be no discrimination between races in the availability of health services.'[34] They also emphasised the need for the government to 'speed up the transition where black and white patients on medical aid can be admitted to hospitals of their choice, African doctors and nurses should be employed in European hospitals.'[35] By 1978, the integration of hospital staff, especially having African nurses practising their craft in white wards or white hospitals, was in full swing across the country. The Provincial Medical Officer of Health of Midlands Province, reported successful efforts at integrating staff and how such a move had averted a disaster. He wrote: 'The integration of African trained staff into the European Hospital, to wards and operating theatres, averted the closure of wards, and this enabled the Hospital to function fully. I am very pleased to say this transition has gone very smoothly. The Sisters [African nursing sisters] have adapted well and have been well received by both patients and staff.'[36] By mid-1978 the gradual approach towards dismantling racial segregation was in progress in other governmental departments.[37] This was partly a result of the shortage of white workers but also as a political need to give a multiracial face to the short-lived Zimbabwe-Rhodesia.

Findings from interviews and newspapers consulted confirm that African nurses were not passive victims of racism and segregation within clinical spaces. They also used the same platform to voice their concerns over unfair treatment and fight for their dignity. During her training as a student nurse at Harari Hospital in the 1970s, Eneresia Makoto remembered staff meetings being tense, often punctuated with intense arguments, with African nurses in more senior positions such as tutors and nursing sisters, at times protesting over unfair treatment of African nurses.[38] She suggested that as much as nothing was done about these complaints, their conduct in meetings was an indicator of their views concerning unjust hospital rules and policies.[39] Besides remonstrations during meetings, given opportunities, African nurses also turned their frustration on white nurses in their everyday work in wards. In 1975, a Select Committee that worked with the Ministry of Health claimed that there were numerous cases of intimidation and discrimination against white student nurses by African tutors at Harari Hospital.[40] These cases were increasing and were an indicator of African nurses' disgruntlement with the system. The Select Committee cited a case of a young white nurse from Rhodesia (born in Rhodesia) who went to Britain for nurse training. When she returned to do her midwifery training in Rhodesia, one of the tutors (African) asked her why she had returned to Rhodesia to do the training. According to the Committee, African nurses told her that the country was not a home for Europeans, it was for blacks and she should have stayed in Britain.[41] The Committee also complained that the same tutors at Harari Hospital insisted on teaching part of their courses in Shona (one of the indigenous languages). When white student nurses indicated that they were unable to follow, African nurses told them that if they wished to live in Zimbabwe, it was time they learned Shona.[42] A year later, in September 1976, the government reported to have conducted extensive and high-powered investigations at Harari and Impilo hospitals on African nurses' supposed misconduct. The allegations centred on the treatment of African members of the Rhodesian Security Forces and freedom fighters. Specifically, African members of the Rhodesian Security Forces were being 'subjected to second-class treatment in certain Rhodesian hospitals. The wounded terrorists (freedom fighters) were treated like heroes by African nurses and orderlies while security forces were given minimum attention.'[43] These complaints were mainly emanating from Impilo and Harari hospitals. Even though Harari and Impilo hospitals were singled out, other hospitals in other districts had one or two such incidents. The Committee failed to prove the validity of the allegations because all the African nurses they quizzed denied the allegations.[44] In February 1977, the newspaper *Property and Finance* maintained the mistreatment of Black Rhodesian Security Forces was continuing, especially at Harari Hospital. The editors wrote:

> The administrators of Harari African Hospital, Salisbury, are concerned at the attitude of certain Black nurses towards wounded Black members of the Security Forces. Some of the wounded [Black members of the Security Force] (it was reported) have been transferred to wards staffed by White nurses. Developments like this would indicate that Black Nationalism, fed on the evidence of weakness (if not surrender) on the part of the Government, is coming more fully into the open.[45]

Again, investigations were fruitless as African nurses denied the allegations. However, interviews confirmed that such cases occasionally occurred. Eneresia Makoto noted that isolated as they might be, such incidents placed nurses in the matrix of the struggle in colonial Zimbabwe. She admitted that whenever they had the chance to nurse wounded guerrillas, they treated them with more respect in comparison to African members of the Rhodesian Security forces. It was, as she argued, their small contribution to the liberation of Zimbabwe, a war they fully supported as 'the boys were fighting to dismantle segregation policies and injustices we experienced every day in colonial Zimbabwe'.[46]

Nursing practice during the war

During the 1970s, urban hospitals experienced a surge in patients visiting. The case of Harari Hospital gives us a good picture of this phenomenon. As the major referral hospital for Africans in the country, the hospital experienced the highest number of patients as patients from rural and urban areas circumvented rural hospitals or council clinics, proceeding directly to Harari. In 1973, the staffing department at Harari expected between 1,500 to 2,000 patients a day seeking treatment, a significant surge as compared to previous years.[47] The Out Patient Department (OPD) was the most affected as an estimated 80 per cent of the patients who sought treatment could have obtained adequate services at clinics in the townships or hospitals in the rural areas.[48] Eneresia Makoto remembers that many patients assumed that they would get the best treatment at Harari, failing to appreciate that township clinics offered similar services.[49] Matrons and other senior personnel complained that high numbers were stretching resources at the referral hospital.[50]

Nurses could not turn away patients as a coping mechanism. It was authorities' obligation to make sure that patients attended the 'right' healthcare centres to spread out the burden between Harari Hospital and council clinics. Hence, it became official policy followed religiously, except in emergency cases that Harari Hospital was to concentrate on cases referred from council clinics and clinics run by commerce and industry.[51] To make sure the public was informed, the government went on a blitz in the press and on the radio, encouraging patients to visit clinics first before turning to referral hospitals. Such an announcement had an immediate impact on nurses working at Harari Central Hospital, as they noticed an almost 90 per cent decline in the number of patients visiting the OPD.[52] This was an ephemeral victory. The intensification of the war in the second half of the decade changed the situation as urban areas experienced an even greater influx of Africans from rural areas. In 1978, the Provincial Medical Officer of Health of Mashonaland Province, was clear on the impact of the war on the provision of health services at Harari Hospital when he wrote: 'The migration of people from rural areas, together with the closure of outlying hospitals and clinics and the disruption of preventative services – all due to the effects of the terrorist activity – has been the main reason for the increased demand of beds ... Staff in all departments have been under pressure and strain. At times the solutions to problems appeared impossible, yet the impossible was always achieved. I am constantly amazed at the resourcefulness of staff and the cheerfulness they display, even in adversity.'[53] The overcrowding at Harari Hospital was also confirmed by the resident doctor, Dr K. A. Beahan, with maternity wards most severely affected. With a capacity of 120 beds, maternity wards were housing up to 190 cases with some expectant mothers sleeping on the floor. As Beahan intimated: 'Our beds are always fully occupied and we are particularly pressed on the maternity side. We have to take room for acute cases and discharge people who are still recovering.'[54] This was just an example of the impact of the war on hospitals. Other hospitals in various urban centres across the country had similar experiences due to war influxes. For example, at Fort Victoria, it was reported that the outpatient attendances at the African Hospital 'increased markedly, especially towards the end of the year, as the result of the closure or partial closure of District Clinics and Chibi Rural Hospital (end of September 1978). Morgenster Mission Hospital, Silvera, St Anton's, Zimutu, Gutu and many Council Clinics are no more'.[55] In the same year, 1978, the Secretary for Health, E. Burnette Smith, admitted that the war had increased the burden on overloaded government hospitals and clinics and curtailed the exploration and control of serious diseases such as bilharzia, malaria and leprosy. In addition, more than 10,000 people suffered from measles in the epidemic that swept through the south-west of the country.[56]

Although Rhodesia's urban healthcare system was under enormous pressure as noted above, it was the rural healthcare system that was mostly affected by the war. Apart from war casualties who became new patients in Rhodesia's hospitals during the 1970s, rural hospitals experienced shortages of medical personnel, widespread intimidation of workers by the warring parties and reduced provision of health services for rural areas. For example, in 1977, the Provincial Medical Officer of Health of Manicaland Province, claimed that in the Rusapi District, various clinics were closed 'with all mission hospitals either closed or working without a doctor's supervision and several doctors in the surrounding districts having had to leave their stations'.[57] In fact, in the previous year (1976), an estimated seventy-one doctors left the country.[58] A significant number of these worked in rural areas and they left partly due to the increased security threats across the country. Besides security threats in rural areas for most medical doctors, junior white doctors skipped the border to avoid military draft.[59] Because of the shortage of military personnel, Rhodesian authorities decreed that all white male doctors under the age of fifty were liable for conscription for up to six months per year.[60] Nurses were also caught up in this ruckus. Though statistics are not available, information from interviews indicates that quite a sizable number of nurses, especially white nurses at rural hospitals, also left the country for their home countries as the war intensified.[61] As with doctors, intimidations from security forces and possibilities of violence played a significant part in compelling nurses to leave the country.[62] Esther Nyanhongo remembers very well in 1977 when Mashoko Mission hospital was closed. All missionary doctors and nurses at the hospital fled the country. The only medical personnel left were African nurses and medical assistants, a situation that forced the main hospital to be closed, especially the main wing. According to Nyanhongo, 'we were now using the hospital mainly as a clinic'.[63] Rural nursing schools were also affected as nurse training schools closed. In 1977 alone, a total of five nursing schools were closed, with two of these being in the war zone province of Manicaland.[64] Mt Selinda Hospital in the southern districts of the province closed in mid-July and Regina Coeli Mission Hospital in the northern parts of the province closed in September 1977, nursing students from the two mission stations being transferred to Umtali.[65] In December 1977, the Matron of the Umtali Nursing School was anticipating more nursing students from another nursing school, Bonda Mission, in January 1978.[66] The closures not only affected nurses' training but also had a huge impact on the communities that had depended on the now closed hospitals for medical services.

Patients in rural areas bore the brunt of these changes. Hospital closures left many without access to medical facilities. To make matters worse, the government rounded up villagers into protected villages in some parts of the country.[67] Many of these protected villages were located far from health centres.[68] Overcrowding and lack of hygiene within protected villages worsened the situation. As E. O'Gorman argued, conditions in protected villages had implications for people's health, especially the very old and young. Within protected villages, there were numerous problems with illnesses such as diarrhoea, scabies and malnutrition.[69] For those who were not dumped into protected villages, the government intensified its surveillance through the imposition of a wartime curfew to control the movement of villagers.[70] As travel was only allowed during the daylight hours, access to medical facilities became limited. E. Nyanhongo explained:

> A pregnant woman needs constant medical attention but being in protected villages and the introduction of curfews in many parts made it more difficult for pregnant mothers to get medical attention. In protected villages, women were usually not allowed to go out without the permission from guards. This meant that even when the time of birth arrives, one had to get clearance/seek permission from the guards to leave. If denied, then one had to give birth at home. Even for those who were not in keeps [protected villages], it was very dangerous to go to hospitals because one risked being shot. Some women had to resort to giving birth at home and it increased the risk of complications and at times death.[71]

It was not only women who were affected by the absence of health facilities. Entire communities found themselves cut off from health centres. In short, hospital closures, protected villages and security risks combined to make it almost impossible for Africans in rural areas to access healthcare, in the process compromising their health.

The dangers posed by the war and the reluctance of medical personnel to call on patients within war zones resulted in making African nurses at rural clinics that were still open the sole authorities on medical issues. In 1976 W. Fraser Ross, of the Department of Social and Preventative Medicine at the University of Rhodesia, observed that the war had induced changes in rural clinics when he wrote that, 'already at a number of rural areas in Rhodesia where formerly a medical practitioner resided, there is a trained nurse endeavouring to carry out some of the functions of the formerly resident doctor'.[72] This type of nurse was called the Advanced Clinical Nurse. Highly trained nurses, the first cohort of nine Advanced Trained Nurses took the course at Impilo Hospital in Bulawayo in 1976. After training they were dispersed throughout the country and 'reports indicate that they have proved a very valuable arm of our Service, and are much appreciated in their respective districts'.[73] The Advanced Clinical Nurse took over the responsibilities of the general practitioner in rural areas they were stationed at.[74] At the outstation clinics that were not covered by the Advanced Clinical Nurses and where medical personnel had stopped or reduced their visits, general nurses became principal authorities in the provision of health services. D. Mtetwa who worked at Chibuwe clinic, recollects:

> During the war, most of us became default authorities especially for those who were working at rural clinics that were still open. Before the war, the medical officer would make weekly visits to each rural clinic under his jurisdiction. The medical officer would see cases we deemed necessary, as well as those that needed to be referred to a larger central district hospital. We would watch him examining the patients, giving us instructions for treatment in case we face similar cases. He would also discuss drug requirements at the clinic and other problems that we might face. At times, he would teach us new practical treatment that he deemed must be introduced at the clinic.[75]

Before the war, nurses were not allowed by the General Medical Officer (GMO)[76] to attend to what were considered as sophisticated cases. Even if it was an emergency, they had to refer such cases to a major hospital. The war, however, altered this rule as the boundary separating the permissible and non-permissible practices of nursing and medicine became blurred. Not only were GMOs unable to attend to patients, for patients themselves, travelling was one of the riskiest affairs. Thus, nurses at some rural clinics in war-torn Rhodesia abrogated the rule as they were left with limited options because of the circumstances they found themselves in:

> We were able to do this [dealing with cases] as we had learnt from training and working with medical doctors. The spectrum of disease we treated was wide generally. It included acute infections, acute malaria, pulmonary disorders, especially pneumonia, bilharzias especially in children and acute disorders. The most common problem was simple wounds and abscesses that we treated with penicillin and other effective remedies. I was lucky not to be confronted with a case that needed surgical services, but I have heard of other nurses who were in such a situation.[77]

The war enabled nurses to expand the scope of nursing practice, asserting their autonomy, and taking responsibility of the rural clinic in the absence of the GMO. As the last bastion of clinical medicine in rural areas, nurses made more decisions than before as they experienced a greater level of autonomy than previously experienced.

The main theatre of war was in the rural areas. Thus, it was mainly Africans residing in rural areas that bore the brunt of the liberation war. They were caught between two armies that were prepared to use any means at their disposal to win the war. Freedom fighters, just as Rhodesian Security Forces, knew that they had to mobilise the full support of the people to win. The rural middle class, such as nurses, teachers, business people, agricultural demonstrators and police, were also caught up in this theatre. As 'middles', nurses used their unique position within rural hospitals to support freedom fighters.[78] Noma Gudhlanga vividly remembered nurses' roles during the liberation war:

> I was working as a nurse at the mission hospital during the war. Nurses, just as teachers, had to provide clothing and other accessories that villagers could not afford to do. As nurses, we were also expected to provide freedom fighters with medicines because we identified with their cause and felt it was our own contribution to the liberation of the country.[79]

Many felt that while they could not hold a gun or directly participate in the war, they had a responsibility to their people and had to support the war in the best way they could. The history of the liberation struggle has mainly been painted in black and white. The study of nurses and the liberation war, however, complicates this narrative. It was not only African nurses who saw it as their responsibility to help freedom fighters with medicine. The solidarity crossed racial divides. Justifiably so, white nurses at mission hospitals could have reported freedom fighters whenever they visited mission hospitals. However, as evidence from literature has shown, they also decided to side with freedom fighters, putting themselves, their staff and the entire mission in harm's way. In her interview with Julie Frederiske, Sr R. Muller remembered her first encounter with freedom fighters, who, *inter alia,* requested medicine from the mission dispensary:

> I said you have to come to the hospital. We don't refuse anybody treatment if they come to the hospital, but we do not give medicine to people because they do not know how to take it, and that is a dangerous thing to just give medicine and then he said, 'oh we do have our own doctor.' Therefore, he called the doctor, he told us the medicines they wanted and we told them the best way was to bring the medicine to them instead.[80]

The above encounter was the first of the many visits to the mission hospital by freedom fighters. Evidence from interviews and literature indicates that once nurses gained freedom fighters' trust, they had to continue working at it lest they be suspected of being informers.[81] Hence, they had to continue their support for freedom fighters, providing them with necessary supplies at requested times. Furthermore, besides giving them medical support, nurses also felt that it was their responsibility to instruct freedom fighters on the best way of using the medicine. Janice McLaughlin notes that at Avila Mission, Mtoko, Sr Josephine, Sr Avila and lay nurses often visited nearby ZANLA (Zimbabwe African National Liberation Army) bases to instruct ZANLA medical officers on how to use medicines.[82] Such a cordial relationship between hospital workers and freedom fighters no doubt cemented the trust between the two groups. At the same time, it is an indicator of how hospital workers also contributed in their respective way to the liberation struggle.

Many nurses at mission hospitals worked as teams to channel medical resources to freedom fighters. They also worked closely with rural villagers in making sure that guerrillas at least had a regular supply of medicines. In her interview with Irene Staunton, Tetty Magugu clearly shows the connection between villagers and nurses and how villagers played an intermediary role in channelling medicine from clinics to guerrillas on behalf of nurses.

> I remember once they asked me to provide them with tablets. I had a friend who worked at the hospital in KweKwe who helped me secure them. Then I had to carry them from town to village. There were often road-blocks where we would be searched and so this was not easy. The way we managed was to cut a hole in the tube of the scotch cart tyre and then we put tablets into it. After that, we mended the tube and inflated it again. That was a clever idea.[83]

The medicines were not destroyed. The success of this mission was an inspiration as she did this several times on her excursion to KweKwe and she found the nurse who worked at KweKwe hospital very generous in providing her with tablets. She continued: 'Generally, whenever I had to go to KweKwe for medicines, I would go by bus. Sometimes we arranged with others from home to meet us in KweKwe and they would travel by scotch cart and, on these occasions, we would put the tube in the cart. Otherwise I would carry it back on bus and pretend that I had taken it to the garage for repair.'[84] Important to appreciate is the networking that took place between nurse and villagers in making medicine available to freedom fighters. In fact, some nurses I talked to have their own stories that are similar to the one cited above. Laiza Shumba sharply recollects her trip to see her parents in a rural area at the height of the war and how she brought medicine for her family which they passed on to freedom fighters:

> My father had been badly beaten up by soldiers [Rhodesian Security Forces] as they suspected that my brother and I had joined the war. In fact, my brother had crossed the border to Zambia but did not join the war. So my sister, who was staying with my parents came and told me how badly injured my father was and what had happened. The hospital in the area had been forced to close and literally, he was stranded. Other villagers were constantly monitoring him so even coming to town would have been difficult if not impossible. My sister managed to leave the village unnoticed. Risking my life, I took medication for my father. I took more than what my father could have used because my sister asked me to bring some for the freedom fighters. I had to bring something for the freedom fighters to show that I supported their cause. Luckily, my sister was nursing her daughter. We had two baby bags and we made sure that we put soiled nappies on top of baby's clothes that covered the medicine. We passed several roadblocks but at one stop, we were searched. They asked me since I was the one carrying the baby. 'What is this?' I said, 'baby clothes.' The white army officer asked me to open it and I did. The moment I opened, the stench came out and he immediately said, '*wena, hamba* (you go)' and that is how I brought the medicine for my father.[85]

She only did this once as she managed to visit her rural home only once in five years. This gesture, passing on medicine to guerrillas, was meant to assure the comrades that her family was not the enemy and they were prepared to do whatever they could if resources were available.

At times nurses were defenceless when security forces visited their areas. They were expected to report any suspicion or presence of freedom fighters. Security forces expected to report suspicious patients, especially unfamiliar faces. In 1970, the failure to report the presence of guerrillas was made a criminal offence, bearing a maximum fine of $600 and/or five years in prison. By 1973, the punishment had escalated to potential life imprisonment.[86] Even such draconian penalties failed to redirect the flow of information to authorities. Although she did not have direct experience with torture or imprisonment at the nearby police camp, Noma Gudhlanga recollected that nurses were just as vulnerable to violence perpetrated by security forces as villagers. Security forces also targeted nurses, claiming nurses were trouble causers in rural areas. Some were arrested on trumped up charges. She recalled how her sister-in-law, who was also a nurse at a rural clinic, was arrested for allegedly aiding guerrillas. She and her six-month-old baby were held for two weeks at the police camp. She was severely tortured.[87] While she acknowledged that nurses aided freedom fighters, Noma Gudhlanga was adamant that in this case her sister-in-law was innocent. She argued, just as what had happened to many innocent civilians who were caught up in the war, these were fabricated charges.[88] Winnie Paradza remembered her ordeal at the hands of the police in the late 1970s:

> The police came to me and said we heard you cooked for the boys and the boys were around here and they were giving politics to you. The first time I refused to talk with them, but later they came with trucks around here and they had to search for everything in the huts. They said, you are the one who gives injections to terrorists because I am working at the mission hospital. The other sister is a European, so they thought that I, as an African, I do everything for the boys. They said, it is better you tell the truth, that you have cooked for the boys and you gave injections to the boys. You just admit it and then you will be freed.[89]

Winnie Paradza's crime, which was in itself a crime punishable by imprisonment, was not only cooking for guerrillas, but also being suspected, as one of the African nurses at the hospital, of supplying freedom fighters with medication. She was beaten up and tortured at Ngundu Police Camp. Her husband experienced the same ordeal when he was accused of aiding her in assisting freedom fighters. They were lucky to be released within a short period.[90] The possibility that Winnie Paradza or Noma Gudhlanga's sister-in-law were in a habit of preparing food for freedom fighters is high. Nurses, just as villagers, made sacrifices to ensure that the war continued. This was part of their contribution to the liberation struggle: providing food and medicines.

The above experiences were usually on an individual and family level. Nurses were also caught up in the crossfire at their workplaces. Clinical spaces became another theatre of struggle as security forces made random, unannounced visits to hospitals, searching for suspected guerrillas or patients who had war wounds. Such visits were also meant to impress upon villagers the dangers of hiding suspected guerrillas or their helpers from government forces. As Noma Gudhlanga claimed:

> As one would expect during the war, there were many tensions between nurses and security forces. Security forces expected us to make reports of any person with war wounds, irrespective of their age. This they meant to use as a way of catching the guerrillas in cases there had been shootings in the area. Patients with war wounds would be arrested as political prisoners and they will be transferred to more secure hospitals in towns. Nurses, like the majority, knew the main reason for the war and we were protective of our people.[91]

Nurses devised methods of protecting themselves from the security forces. For example, if they had a patient with what was suspected as war wounds, they changed records and used pseudonyms to protect the patient or their families in the village. It was not that security forces would read diagnosis records, but this survival mechanism was a protection measure in case soldiers suspected someone. Besides falsifying records and names, nurses would also hide patients that might be in trouble from security forces by making them sleep next to other patients and covering them when security forces came.[92] While in most cases nurses were threatened with imprisonment if they failed to cooperate, at times security officers threatened them with death. In her study on Catholic Missions during the war, Janice McLaughlin argues that nurses at mission hospitals were in a precarious position vis-à-vis the security forces.[93] At Avila Mission, Mtoko District, one of the nurses, Ephiphania Nyandoro, recalled when Rhodesian soldiers came to the clinic searching for injured ZANLA guerrillas.[94] Security beat the nurses, threatened to close the clinic and to kill the most senior nurse at the hospital, Sr Josephine. Violence and intimidation of nursing personnel by security forces aimed to make sure that nurses cooperated. According to Ephiphania Nyandoro, that night, Sr Josephine slept in the clinic with patients as the soldiers were constantly monitoring movements at the convent.[95] Sr Josephine survived her ordeal. Important to appreciate is that many nurses found themselves in the crossfire during the war. Just as rural villagers suffered the harshness of the war, the rural nurse not only contributed through provision of food, clothing and money, but also used her position within clinical spaces to make medicine available to freedom fighters. Additionally, rural nurses also used clinical spaces to shelter victims who might have been at the mercy of the security forces. In nursing the nation at war, the rural nurse received death threats and at times paid a heavy price that included torture and beatings.

Healthcare work within the war zones

Some trained medical and nursing personnel left Rhodesia to join up with the liberation forces to fight for Zimbabwe's independence. The ZANU medical department had medical doctors such as Herbert Ushewokunze, Sydney Sekeramayi and Felix Muchemwa.[96] In the case of ZAPU, medical doctors Gordon Bango and Benjamin Dube were in charge of health facilities in ZIPRA bases as well as refugee camps.[97] ZAPU was based in Zambia. Mavhunga noted that before 1979, ZAPU did not have any field hospitals and thus relied on the medical facilities made available by the Zambian Government, such as the University Teaching Hospital in Lusaka, and other government medical facilities in Kabwe, the Copperbelt, Kitwe and Ndola.[98] With the intensification of the war, together with the increase in medical personnel, by 1979 they had a mobile hospital and two field hospitals based at Solowezi and Victoria camps. The two field hospitals had a capacity of 250 beds.[99] In the case of ZANU, while they also relied on Mozambican facilities such as the Chimoio Hospital, they also had their field hospitals that catered for combatants and refugees alike. Named after the first African medical doctor in Rhodesia and a nationalist of the liberation struggle, Dr Samuel Parirenyatwa, the Parirenyatwa Bush Hospital had at least 100 beds. It was a makeshift hospital. The wards were constructed mainly of wood and grass and the medical workers used a tent as a theatre. They referred critical cases to Mozambican hospitals. The hospital had three mobile operating units on wheels and three ambulances.[100]

Marjorie Makaza was clear, for such hospitals to function well in such a hostile environment with limited resources, they had to work as a team. She noted, 'while we maintained the ordinary structures of medical facilities, team work was significant. We were a full-fledged team'.[101] What Makaza emphasised, which is a running theme of their work, was the significance of workers other than medical doctors in the functioning of these hospitals. The burden of treating the wounded and nursing the infirm – combatants and refugees alike – lay on the shoulders of a host of a broad range of healthcare workers who included nurses, nursing assistants and medics. The nurses and medics had three roles: fighting to defend themselves, fighting the Rhodesian security forces, in addition to ensuring sound health for the guerrilla fighters and refugees. In other words, they fought diseases as much as they fought the enemy.[102] Some of the healthcare workers had prior education in nursing and medicine and had worked in Rhodesian hospitals before they joined the war. The cases of Getrude Mutasa and Marjorie Makaza immediately come to mind. Born in 1946 in the Chikomba District, Mutasa did her nurse internship at Harari Hospital before going to England for further training. She stressed, 'While in England, we had seen the bombing going on back home, and one would only be moved to come and help.'[103] She narrated that: 'In 1977, the liberation struggle had intensified, and ZANLA (Zimbabwe African National Liberation Army) saw the dire need to recruit additional medical personnel to help casualties at the battle front.'[104] Thus, moved by her compassion to help the suffering, she relocated to Mozambique. With her nursing experience, the authorities appointed her the medical officer for ZANLA headquarters in Maputo. She was responsible for receiving, screening, treating and referring injured fighters from the war front, especially in the Gaza province.[105] Marjorie Makaza did not join the war via England. Her journey was slightly different but like Mutasa, her role, and that of her colleagues was to ensure that the patients – combatants and refugees – lived.[106] Born in Sakubva Township, Umtali, Marjorie Makaza did her fist two years of nursing at Umtali Hospital until she left for Mozambique:

> We would read in newspapers on what was going on in the country. At the end of the first year of our nursing school, my friend and I began contemplating joining the war. We were not into politics, but we had a feeling that we must do something. Initially, we thought we would serve our people when we completed our studies. Then in our second year, we had a weekend off. We went to visit our parents in the township and we never went back to the nursing school. With other two young men and women, we skipped

the country. We could have used the route popularised by migrants who traversed Zimbabwe and Mozambique, but we thought it was dangerous. Hence, we had to navigate the mined border between Zimbabwe and Mozambique. After crossing into Mozambique, we were introduced to other comrades, who also referred us to others and we transferred to the refugee camp where we were vetted.[107]

The vetting processes included a comprehensive and at times exhaustive interrogation and a medical check-up to determine suitability for military training. They assigned other tasks to those considered unsuitable for military training. According to Makaza,

> All along, I had not mentioned that I had trained as a nurse even though I did not complete the programme. It was during the medical examination that I revealed this information. The medic, comrade Tichapfuma stared at me and more or less interrogated me about aspects of medical practices, nursing and general public health. Satisfied, he instructed me to leave. After a few days, we commenced our military training but by then I was told that I will be useful in the medical department.[108]

Makaza and Mutasa are emblematical of those with experience in nursing and medical practices. However, some who later on provided nursing as well as medical services to their colleagues and in some cases, the general populace in the camps, had no prior knowledge of medicine and nursing. Because of difficulty in recruiting qualified people to work within the medical departments and of course the circumstances, they had to forgo some of the established protocols of training nurses and orderlies in Rhodesia. For example, in Rhodesia, for one to become an orderly or a nurse, they must have reached a certain level of education. Makaza remarked 'this was wartime and in a war zone. Some of the conditions that were emphasised if one wanted to become a nurse were not adhered.'[109] Quite a number of these men and women were 'trained on the job.'[110]

Before being chosen to concentrate on the medical aspects of the war, combatants had to go for military training. The training lasted for at least six months. Those who had done well or showed promise in medical aid courses were recruited to go further in nursing and other aspects of medicine. Makaza remarked: 'It made sense to encourage the ones who were doing well in aspects of health. They would have shown their potential within this field.'[111] Their training focused on general nursing and medical practices. It was geared towards teaching the recruits the nature of medical and health problems they were likely to encounter at the 'rear' – that is the refugee camps and operational bases within the host countries of Mozambique and Zambia, as well as the 'war front' – that is the theatre of war inside Rhodesia. Aspects of public health focused on maintaining good health in the base camps and refugee camps.[112] For the most part, the provision of health services in camps was rudimentary.[113] Cases of waterborne diseases, especially dysentery, diarrhoea and cholera, were common. Scholars agree that the Rhodesian security forces, especially the Selous Scouts, used cholera as one of their biological weapons. They planted the cholera bacterium into water reservoirs and guerrillas 'leaving for the front or to conduct other errands that spread the bacterium over a wide arc'.[114] Besides waterborne diseases, there were high incidences of malnutrition. Akwino Aquous Muwoni stated that 'we had many cases of food related diseases and some deficiencies due to lack of proper diet'.[115] There were cases of sexually transmitted infections, but as Muchemwa highlighted, they were rare: 'I have never treated any comrade for an STI from the front but here and there at the rear. It is not surprising that there were no cases of STI from the front. You see, the medics who were at the front were so knowledgeable about STIs. They would inject themselves.'[116] In his interview, Muchemwa did not indicate why there were fewer cases of STIs at the front. It is likely that Muchemwa wanted to present an image of disciplined and dedicated cadres.[117] Marjorie Makaza indicated that due to the nature of the operations, guerrillas had less time to engage in sexual relations when at the front, thus reducing the chances of the spread of STIs.[118] Whether they were at the battle front or the rear, STIs were one of the health problems guerrilla medics and nurses dealt with.

The theatre of war was on the front – inside Rhodesia. While mission hospitals in Rhodesia at times aided the guerrillas as noted in the previous section, this was an exception to the rule. Each guerrilla unit had a medic and the medic was knowledgeable and could treat any condition befalling members of the unit. Thus, while their training focused on general public health, more importantly, it emphasised the treatment of injured combatants in the field. For those who had prior knowledge of nursing, this was totally new. Makaza remembered that: 'My nursing education did not include aspects of treatment related to war injuries. Learning how to treat war injuries was new to me.'[119] Akwino Aquous Muwoni, a medic during the war, highlighted that:

> We learnt to treat gunshot wounds, bomb injuries inflicted by shrapnel, studied chemical warfare and how to contain it, we studied how to deal with food poisoning, the poisoning of clothes and water poisoning ... the enemy also used napalm bombs, it would 'eat' one's body in a few minutes. We were also trained that even after heavy battle with some casualties we were never supposed to leave injured comrades. This was because the injured comrade once captured would be tortured and forced to reveal all training programmes and camps. Once a comrade was injured in a battle, the medical corps was supposed to take command and ensure the comrade survives.[120]

There were no clinics, hospitals or ambulances in the war zone: 'but we had the best kit in the form of medicine ... [medical kit] others were given grenades, bombs etc. but my equipment was the medical kit'.[121] On the front, therefore, while the rest of the members of each fighting unit had guns and other weapons of war, guerrilla medics had their weapon – the medical kit. They played their fair share in alleviating suffering amongst their comrades.

The war was fought on an unequal footing. Rhodesian security forces had an array of resources at their disposal. Guerrillas had limited resources, which presented challenges to guerrilla medical units. Worse for the guerrillas, the Rhodesians also relied on biological warfare in their efforts to contain guerrilla incursions into Rhodesia. Ian Martinez demonstrated that by the late 1970s, the Rhodesians resorted to the use of bacteriological and chemical weapons as 'dirty tricks'. In the process, they employed different techniques that included poisoning wells, spreading cholera, infecting clothing and using anthrax to kill cattle, thus denying food supplies to guerrillas.[122] At one time, Chief Medical Officer at the bush hospital, Parirenyatwa Hospital, Dr Felix Muchemwa narrated how he was moved to a base in Mozambique by the ZANLA commander, Gn. Josiah Tongogara, due to the problems they were experiencing as a result of the Rhodesian biological warfare:

> he [Tongogara] told me that they were having problems at the front. He said there were some drugs that were being used against the comrades by the Smith regime. He said some of the drugs were being put in their clothing, especially jeans, shirts and even underpants that would be looking new. He

said after putting on these clothes many comrades would just be sweating, start being restless and collapse. There was also organophosphorus compound poisoning, especially Malathion. This was used to contaminate mainly clothes. The other chemicals the Rhodesians used included cyanide, thallium which they would inject into injectable drugs like antibiotics. The moment we treated our comrades using contaminated drugs, the comrades would just collapse. Sometimes we would think that fellow comrades are killing each other when actually the drugs were contaminated. These contaminated drugs would be distributed to most mission clinics and hospitals especially rural clinics. The worst was food poisoning. Tinned beef, tinned beans, anything tinned the Rhodesians would put thallium which is the highest poison in the world.[123]

The types of clothing treated with poison included underpants, t-shirts and denim jeans.[124] Denims were part of the regalia popular with guerrillas because they lasted longer.[125] Besides tinned foods, the Rhodesians contaminated mealie meal and beer with thallium and poisoned cartons of cigarettes with toxins. In 1978, the Rhodesian Commissioner of Police, Peter Allum, gave an order to Rhodesian security forces to stop all covert poisoning operations.[126] However, the manufacture and spread of poison by the Rhodesian forces continued into mid-1979.[127] As Muchemwa pointed out above, to some extent, it achieved some success. For the medics and nurses, chemical warfare added another layer to the challenges they faced. Mutasa summarised the challenges that were brought on by the use of chemical weapons in the daily work of nurses during the war. She highlighted that their experiences with victims of chemical warfare almost made conventional hospital work a stroll in the park; 'such antics [the use of chemicals] resulted in the victims developing sores in the alimentary canal, while others lost their voices as a result. The situation posed a complex challenge to the freedom fighters, as most of the ailments lacked pharmaceutical remedies.'[128] In response, the medical units began training the medics and other healthcare workers on biological warfare.[129]

In their various capacities – either as nurses or as medics – and either at the warfront or at the rear base, guerrilla healthcare workers had to be creative in the ways they provided nursing and medical services to their patients. An example of being inventive in the provision of surgical services was the bush theatres. At Parirenyatwa Hospital, they did not perform surgical operations within the premises of the hospital. Rather, they established bush theatres using tents at a distance from the hospital. According to Muwoni: 'We had opportunities of having some surgical operations that we undertook in the bush. We would go out of the camp complex where we would establish bush theatres using tents ... These theatres were disinfected, and they were like normal theatres. This is where we would take injured comrades and operated on them with the assistance from doctors.'[130] The surgeries took place during the day and the patients were transferred to the wards at night. There were cases where they evacuated entire wards during the day and patients were transported back into the wards at night. Their medical and nursing needs were taken care of outside the hospital. In addition, food for the patients would be prepared in the camps and then brought to the patients outside the camps.[131] This was to protect patients in case of attacks, especially aerial attacks from the Rhodesian security forces.

Besides being creative in performing medical operations, at times wartime surgeries enabled medics and nurses to encroach into medical practice. Often, medics and nurses performed minor surgeries, in the process blurring the boundaries between medical and nursing practices. As in some rural hospitals noted earlier, the occasional absence of a medical doctor left the nurse/orderly with no choice but to execute tasks normally reserved for medical doctors. The case of Muwoni illustrates this. As he narrated, he and Dr Sekeramayi had prepared a theatre procedure to operate on an injured combatant who had a foreign body within the testicle. Just before they began, General Josiah Tongagara, the ZANLA commander, called Sekeramayi. Sekeremayi left Muwoni to carry out the operation. Muwoni stated that, 'I had handed the surgical blade over to Dr Sekeramayi, but when this call came he gave me back the blade and instructed me to continue with the delicate operation.' Sekeramayi had performed several operations with Muwoni, hence his confidence in Muwoni's abilities. Following instructions, Muwoni managed to remove the foreign body, cleaned the opening with an antiseptic and completed the operation without any problems. According to Muwoni, 'this was my first operation on such a delicate organ of the human body'.[132] Nicknamed 'the bush doctor' for the operation, it is possible that this was not the last operation he executed.

There was also creativity on the warfront. Guerrillas operated in sections of plus or minus ten – consisting of a commander, a political commissar, a security logistics officer, three to five cadres and a medical officer. Besides being armed, the medic also carried a medical kit as previously noted. Akwino Aquous Muwoni claimed that medical kits would have 'strong painkillers, antibiotics, anaesthesics and surgical instruments for minor operations',[133] but Rhodesian medical officers claimed that the medical kits from captured guerrillas consisted of 'dirty disposable syringes (used many times and never cleaned), some sulfa drugs, frequently penicillin and anti-malarials, but always fair quantities of cannabis (dagga)'.[134] Irrespective of the different descriptions of the medical kit contents, important to highlight is that the guerrilla medics worked with limited resources. Worse, at times, medics encountered medical problems beyond their scope. In case of complex medical situations, they sometimes resorted to sympathetic mission clinics or hospitals as already noted. The medics ensured that the wounded reached the mission station. Failure to access mission hospitals resulted in long journeys back to the base camp with injured cadres. In all cases, the evacuations of the wounded required innovation. Muwoni's experiences give us a rough picture of not only the paucity of resources available to medics, but also of the ways in which they were resourceful when it came to evacuating injured combatants from the warfront to the rear. A medic himself, Muwoni was injured following an attack at the warfront. During retreating from the battle, they lost their medical kit, leaving Muwoni and his colleagues without medical supplies. Losing a lot of blood, his fellow combatants took him to the 'base' where some people at the 'base', 'prepared thin porridge for me to drink so that I can regain my energy'.[135] Within the indigenous nursing practices, thin porridge (*usvusvu*) is given to patients as the first step towards recuperation. Without their medical kit, the combatants had to find other ways of ensuring that their colleague survived the ordeal. Using the few available resources, Muwoni's colleagues tore bed sheets into bandages and prepared a makeshift stretcher using planks and sacks.[136] As Muwoni emphasised, 'this makeshift stretcher was also an ambulance during the liberation struggle'.[137] At times, the combatants used bicycles as an 'ambulance to transport injured comrades'.[138] In this event, however, they had no other option but to use the makeshift stretcher to transport the injured Muwoni from the warfront to the rear. He recounted that: 'So, my ambulance was quickly constructed, and we started the evacuation exercise from Matibi 31 area. The people carried me on a stretcher and we started walking back to Chicualacuala.'[139] It took them at least six days to travel to their destination. To avoid detection, they travelled at night and rested under cover during the day. Muwoni continued, 'I was the expert in medicine, but now I was on the stretcher writhing in pain.'[140] After reaching Mozambique, Muwoni was admitted at Barrage Military Hospital where doctors operated on him and removed a foreign body. Later on, he discovered that he had another foreign object lodged in his shoulder.[141] Muwoni lived to narrate his ordeal but others did not. In the heat of crossfire, at times the combatants left their wounded colleagues in the battlefield to die a slow and agonising death.[142] Significant to appreciate here is the ingenuity of medics and their colleagues in alleviating suffering considering the limited resources they had at their disposal.

The experiences of healthcare workers such as Mutasa, Muwoni and Makaza are emblematical of the experiences of many medics during the war. The syringe was their gun.[143] With the coming of independence in 1980, they were reintegrated into society as with other combatants. Makaza completed her nursing degree and later on specialised in the rehabilitation of combatants. Mutasa initially joined Harari Hospital as nurse and later on joined to the Zimbabwe National Army. Besides holding various army ranks, she also served as the medical and training staff officer, chief nursing officer and deputy director of the army medical services. Muwoni also assisted in integrating the different fighting forces into one army, the Zimbabwe National Army. He later on furthered his education and did a number of postgraduate courses within the health profession, specialising in midwifery, general nursing, dentistry, the management of malaria, and family planning.

Conclusion

The decade of the 1970s brought new challenges within Rhodesian society. The tensions that had simmered for a long time blew into a war by the beginning of 1972. The war lasted until 1979. Within this environment, Rhodesian hospitals became another site of struggle for the racial acrimony that was being played out outside of the walls of hospitals. Thus, one finds in the 1970s a sustained criticism from blacks and liberal whites against some of the hospital policies that emphasised limited contact between whites and blacks in Rhodesian government hospitals. In all this, the role of African nurses inside Rhodesian hospitals took centre stage, particularly whether the African nurse could work in white wards or not. During a time when hospitals had closed some white wards due to the shortage of white nurses to take care of white patients, a significant number of black nurses were failing to secure employment. However, the policy was contradictory considering that African domestic workers sustained white households throughout the colonial period. Furthermore, as pointed out by Levy and African legislators, at times, whites resorted to using equipment in African hospitals or even consulted African doctors as the case of Dr Mzengezi illustrated. With the intensification of war and the increase in white staff attrition, and as part of the efforts to appease internal nationalists, the government began to turn a blind eye on the policy that restricted African nurses' presence within white hospitals.

The war affected nurses in various ways. During the war, rural dwellers fled the countryside seeking refuge in urban areas. Increased urbanisation stretched hospital resources and affected the provision of nursing services, leaving nurses in urban hospitals with increased workloads. As with earlier generations of nurses, nurses working in urban areas used various strategies to lessen the strain of providing services to an increased number of patients with limited resources. However, it was rural nurses who had the most unenviable tasks. Providing hospital services in a war-torn countryside came with its dangers. Caught in the middle of two warring armies, African nurses did not abandon their rural posts. Instead, they provided services even though they put their lives at risks. The nurses contended that the provision of hospital services in the war-torn countryside constituted their contribution to the emancipation of the nation. While rural nurses had their fair share of problems, juggling between two belligerent forces, the medics and other healthcare workers who provided medical and nursing services to combatants fighting for the liberation of Zimbabwe provided services with limited resources. While some of them had nursing and medical training before joining the war, the majority of these had limited nursing and medical experience as they trained on the job. As with the earlier generation of nurses that was central to the provision of health services to Africans in rural areas, the medic became the bastion of the bush hospital. It can be argued that the 1970s war transformed nurses' work environment, so that by the end of the war, African nurses were officially nursing whites and, irrespective of the hospital they worked in, they dealt with nursing and medical problems inflicted by the war. The coming of independence in 1980 and the policies put into place by the post-colonial government, together with the changing disease environment, would bring other changes and challenges to Zimbabwean hospitals and nurses' everyday work.

Notes

1 Report of the Secretary for Health for the year ending 31 December 1978.
2 See *Property and Finance*, May 1971 and June 1971.
3 Report of the Secretary for Health for the year ending 31 December 1974.
4 Report of the Secretary for Health for the year ending 31 December 1974.
5 NAZ MS 308/82/2, Health Services in Relation to the Liberation Struggle, newspaper cutting from *The Rhodesia Herald*, 25 January 1975.
6 NAZ MS 308/82/2, Health Services in Relation to the Liberation Struggle, newspaper cutting from *The Rhodesia Herald*, 25 January 1975.
7 *The Rhodesia Herald*, 21 November 1974.
8 *The Rhodesia Herald*, 22 January 1975.
9 *The Rhodesia Herald*, 25 January 1975.
10 *The Rhodesia Herald*, 25 January 1975.
11 *The Rhodesia Herald*, 22 January 1975.
12 L. F. Levy, 'Keeping abreast of the times', *Central African Journal of Medicine*, 8: 2 (1962), pp. 158–9.
13 NAZ MS 308/38/2 Health Services in Relation to the Liberation Struggle, newspaper cutting from *The Rhodesia Herald*, 22 January 1975.
14 NAZ MS 308/38/2 Health Services in Relation to the Liberation Struggle.
15 J. Whitehead, 'The Andrew Fleming Hospital, Salisbury, Rhodesia', *Annals of the Royal College of Surgeons of England*, 54 (1974), pp. 313–14.
16 Whitehead, 'The Andrew Fleming Hospital, Salisbury'.
17 Interview: Mrs Matondo, Sakubva Mutare, 12 August 2008.
18 NAZ MS 308/38/2 Health Services in Relation to the Liberation Struggle, newspaper cutting from *The Rhodesia Herald*, 22 January 1975.

19 NAZ MS 308/38/2 Health Services in Relation to the Liberation Struggle, newspaper cutting from *The Rhodesia Herald*, 25 January 1975.
20 Interview: Mrs Matondo, Sakubva Mutare, 12 August 2008.
21 The Land Apportionment Act (1930) was the most comprehensive legislation dealing on the land issue. This Act became the hallmark of Rhodesian society meant to stave off racial competition. It demarcated land between races. Africans could not buy land or lease property within white areas, hence the special instruction from the Minister to allow Dr Mzengezi to lease property in the white section of Gwelo.
22 NAZ MS 308/38/2 Health Services in Relation to the Liberation Struggle, newspaper cutting from *The Rhodesia Herald*, 21 November 1974.
23 NAZ MS 308/38/2 Health Services in Relation to the Liberation Struggle, newspaper cutting from *The Rhodesia Herald*, 21 November 1974.
24 None of my interviewees worked in the private sector. Nevertheless, they reiterated that African doctors who had private surgeries employed African nurses.
25 Marks, *Divided sisterhood*, pp. 189–93.
26 NAZ MS 308/38/2 Health Services in Relation to the Liberation Struggle, newspaper cutting from *The Rhodesia Herald*, 22 January 1975.
27 R. T. D. Sadomba, *Rhodesia Parliamentary Debates*, vol. 91, 5–29 August 1975.
28 R. T. D. Sadomba, *Rhodesia Parliamentary Debates*, vol. 91, 5–29 August 1975.
29 NAZ MS 308/38/2 Health Services in Relation to the Liberation Struggle.
30 Interview: Mrs Nelia Ncube, Chitungwiza, 20 April 2009.
31 Dr Barlow, *Rhodesia Parliamentary Debates*, vol. 91, 5–29 August 1975.
32 Report of the Secretary for Health for the year ending 31 December 1976.
33 Report of the Secretary for Health for the year ending 31 December 1976.
34 NAZ MS 308/38/3 Health Services in Relation to the Liberation Struggle, newspaper cutting from *The Rhodesia Herald*, 24 September 1977.
35 NAZ MS 308/38/3 Health Services in Relation to the Liberation Struggle, newspaper cutting from *The Rhodesia Herald*, 24 September 1977.
36 Report of the Secretary for Health for the year ending 31 December 1978.
37 For other government departments such as the army, see for example, T. Stapleton, *African police and soldiers in colonial Zimbabwe, 1923–1980* (Rochester, NY: University of Rochester Press, 2011) pp. 183–4.
38 Interview: Mrs Eneresia Makoto, Harare, 28 January 2009.
39 Interview: Mrs Eneresia Makoto, Harare, 28 January 2009.
40 Dr Barlow, Rhodesia Parliamentary Debates, vol. 91, 5–29 August 1975.
41 Dr Barlow, Rhodesia Parliamentary Debates, vol. 91, 5–29 August 1975.
42 Dr Barlow, Rhodesia Parliamentary Debates, vol. 91, 5–29 August 1975.
43 NAZ MS 308/38/2 Health Services in Relation to the Liberation Struggle, newspaper cutting from *Rhodesian Financial Gazette*, 10 September 1976.
44 NAZ MS 308/38/2 Health Services in Relation to the Liberation Struggle, newspaper cutting from *Rhodesian Financial Gazette*, 10 September 1976.

45 *Property and Finance*, February 1977, 'Black nurses and the wounded'.
46 Interview: Mrs Eneresia Makoto, Harare, 28 January 2009.
47 NAZ MS 308/38/1 Health Services in Relation to the Liberation Struggle, newspaper cutting from *The Rhodesia Herald*, 6 April 1973.
48 Interview: Mrs Eneresia Makoto, Harare, 28 January 2009.
49 Interview: Mrs Eneresia Makoto, Harare, 28 January 2009.
50 NAZ MS 308/38/1 Health Services in Relation to the Liberation Struggle.
51 NAZ MS 308/38/1 Health Services in Relation to the Liberation Struggle, cutting from *Moto*, 30 June 1973.
52 NAZ MS 308/38/1 Health Services in Relation to the Liberation Struggle, cutting from *Moto*, 30 June 1973.
53 Report of the Secretary for Health for the year ending 31 December 1978.
54 NAZ MS 308/38/4 Health Services in Relation to the Liberation Struggle, newspaper cutting from *The National Observer*, 28 December 1978.
55 Report of the Secretary for Health for the year ending 31 December 1978.
56 NAZ MS 308/38/4 Health Services in Relation to the Liberation Struggle, the Health Secretary's Report of 1977 quoted in the British Broadcasting report, 6 October 1978.
57 Report of the Secretary for Health for the year ending 31 December 1977.
58 NAZ MS 308/38/3 Health Services in Relation to the Liberation Struggle, report by Sue Challis, 'When medical care becomes a weapon', 19 November 1977.
59 NAZ MS 308/38/3 Health Services in Relation to the Liberation Struggle.
60 According to Wilkinson, the average monthly net outflow was 13,709 in 1978. This was the highest in the country's history. For more see A. R. Wilkinson, 'The impact of the war', in W. H. Morris-Jones, *From Rhodesia to Zimbabwe: Behind and beyond Lancaster House* (London: Frank Cass, 1980), pp. 110–23.
61 Interview: Mrs Esther Nyanhongo, Harare, 28 January 2009.
62 Besides the provision of basic health care services being affected, education services were also affected by the war. *The Rhodesia Herald* reported that by November 1978, 951 primary schools had closed, leaving more than 230,000 children without schooling (about 25 per cent of the total) as a result of the war. Thirty-five secondary schools and their 9,000 pupils were similarly affected. Over 2,000 teachers had lost their jobs. See *The Rhodesia Herald*, 22 November 1978.
63 Interview: Mrs Esther Nyanhongo, Harare, 28 January 2009.
64 NAZ MS 308/38/3 Health Services in Relation to the Liberation Struggle, newspaper cutting from *The Rhodesia Herald*, 1 October 1977 and Report of the Secretary for Health for the year ending 31 December 1977.
65 Report of the Secretary for Health for the year ending 31 December 1977.
66 Report of the Secretary for Health for the year ending 31 December 1977.

67 Protected villages were forms of concentration camps, established from 1974, where peasants were forced to live behind a fence from where their every movement was monitored by guard forces.
68 For a comprehensive study on protected villages, see for example, E. O'Gorman, *The front line runs through every woman: Women and local resistance in the Zimbabwean War* (London: James Currey, 2011).
69 O'Gorman, *The front line runs*, pp. 94–5.
70 O'Gorman, *The front line runs*, pp. 94–5.
71 Interview: Mrs Esther Nyanhongo, Harare, 28 January 2009.
72 W. Fraser Ross, 'The Advanced Clinical Nurse', *Central African Journal of Medicine*, 22: 3 (1976), p. 56.
73 Report of the Secretary for Health for the year ending 31 December 1978.
74 W. Fraser Ross, 'The Advanced Clinical Nurse', p. 56.
75 Interview: Mrs D. Mtetwa, Mutare, August 2008.
76 The principal medical officer responsible for a district.
77 Interview: Mrs D. Mtetwa, Mutare, August 2008.
78 Interview: Mrs Noma Gudhlanga, Mutare, 28 August 2008.
79 Interview: Mrs Noma Gudhlanga, Mutare, 28 August 2008.
80 Sr R. Muller quoted in J. Frederikse, *None but ourselves: Masses and media in the making of Zimbabwe* (New York: Penguin Books, 1984), pp. 302–3.
81 Interview: Mrs Shumba, Mabelreign Harare, 26 October 2008.
82 J. McLaughlin, *On the frontline: Catholic missions in Zimbabwe liberation war* (Baobab Books: Harare, 1996), p. 201.
83 Tetty Magugu, Zhombe, Interview in I. Staunton (ed.), *Mothers of the revolution: The war experiences of thirty Zimbabwean women* (London: James Currey, 1990), p. 161.
84 Tetty Magugu, Interview in Staunton (ed.), *Mothers of the revolution*, p. 161.
85 Interview: Mrs Shumba, Mabelreign Harare, 26 October 2008.
86 Frederikse, *None but ourselves*, p. 83.
87 Interview: Mrs Noma Gudhlanga, Mutare, 28 August 2008.
88 Interview: Mrs Noma Gudhlanga, Mutare, 28 August 2008.
89 Winnie Paradza quoted in Frederikse, *None but ourselves*, pp. 72–3.
90 Winnie Paradza quoted in Frederikse, *None but ourselves*, pp. 72–3.
91 Interview: Mrs Noma Gudhlanga, Mutare, 28 August 2008.
92 Interview: Mrs Noma Gudhlanga, Mutare, 28 August 2008.
93 McLaughlin, *On the frontline*, p. 82.
94 Zimbabwe African National Liberation Army (ZANLA) was the armed wing of Zimbabwe African Nation Union Patriotic Front (ZANU PF), one of the liberation struggle movements.
95 Epiphania Nyandoro quoted in McLaughlin, *On the frontline*, p. 83.
96 Interview: Brig. Felix Muchemwa, *The Sunday Mail*, 17–23 March 2013. Interview by M. Huni.

97 C. C. Mavhunga, 'Guerrilla healthcare innovation: Creative resilience in Zimbabwe's Chimurenga, 1971–1980', *History and Technology*, 31: 3 (2015), p. 301.
98 Mavhunga, 'Guerrilla healthcare innovation', p. 299.
99 Mavhunga, 'Guerrilla healthcare innovation', p. 300.
100 Mavhunga, 'Guerrilla healthcare innovation', p. 302.
101 Interview: Marjorie M. Makaza, Mutare, 17 April 2015.
102 Interview: Marjorie M. Makaza, Mutare, 17 April 2015.
103 Interview: Brig. Gertrude Mutasa, *The Sunday Mail*, 11–16 February 2007. Interview by M. Mkwate.
104 Interview: Brig. Gertrude Mutasa, *The Sunday Mail*, 11–16 February 2007. Interview by M. Mkwate.
105 *The Herald*, 7 October 2013.
106 Interview: Marjorie M. Makaza, Mutare, 17 April 2015.
107 Interview: Marjorie M. Makaza, Mutare, 17 April 2015.
108 Interview: Marjorie M. Makaza, Mutare, 17 April 2015.
109 Interview: Marjorie M. Makaza, Mutare, 17 April 2015.
110 Interview: Akwino Aquous Muwoni, aka Texan Chidhakwa, *The Sunday Mail*, 5–11 May 2013. Interview by M. Huni.
111 Interview: Marjorie M. Makaza, Mutare, 17 April 2015.
112 Interview: Marjorie M. Makaza, Mutare, 17 April 2015.
113 In 1977, the Medical Officer at Chipinga Hospital claimed that the captured wounded guerrillas repeatedly said that very many recruits had died of disease or from accidents in their training camps in Mozambique, where medical treatment was rudimentary. Report of the Secretary for Health for the year ending 31 December 1977.
114 Mavhunga, 'Guerrilla healthcare innovation', p. 310.
115 Interview: Akwino Aquous Muwoni, aka Texan Chidhakwa, *The Sunday Mail*, 5–11 May 2013. Interview by M. Huni.
116 Interview: Brig. Felix Muchemwa, *The Sunday Mail*, 17–23 March 2013. Interview by M. Huni.
117 It is also possible that Muchemwa was responding to Rhodesian propaganda that presented guerrillas as purveyors of STIs. See, Catholic Commission for Justice and Peace, *Rhodesia: The propaganda war: Report prepared by the members of the Commission for Justice and Peace inside Rhodesia* (London: The Catholic Institute for International Relations, 1977), p. 8.
118 Interview: Marjorie M. Makaza, Mutare, 17 April 2015. It must be pointed out that guerrillas were at times involved in sexual relations when at the front. And Rhodas Karimakwenda's interview revealed that there was rampant sexual abuse at the rear – in the camps and refugee camps. See Rhodas Karimakwenda (nom de guerre – Anna Matambudziko), *The Sunday Mail*, 26 January – 1 February 2020. Interview by N. Muchemwa.
119 Interview: Marjorie M. Makaza, Mutare, 17 April 2015.

120 Interview: Akwino Aquous Muwoni, aka Texan Chidhakwa, *The Sunday Mail*, 5–11 May 2013. Interview by M. Huni.
121 Interview: Akwino Aquous Muwoni, aka Texan Chidhakwa, *The Sunday Mail*, 5–11 May 2013. Interview by M. Huni.
122 I. Martinez, 'The history of the use of bacteriological and chemical agents during Zimbabwe's liberation war of 1965–80 by Rhodesian forces', *Third World Quarterly*, 23: 6, 2002, pp. 1163–4.
123 Interview: Brig. Felix Muchemwa, *The Sunday Mail*, 17–23 March 2013. Interview by M. Huni.
124 P. L. Moorcroft and P. McLaughlin, *The Rhodesian war: Fifty years on* (South Yorkshire: Pen and Sword Books Ltd, 2015), p. 106.
125 Interview: Marjorie M. Makaza, Mutare, 17 April 2015.
126 Moorcroft and McLaughlin, *The Rhodesian war*, p. 106.
127 Moorcroft and McLaughlin, *The Rhodesian war*, p. 106.
128 Interview: Brig. Gertrude Mutasa, *The Sunday Mail*, 11–16 February 2007. Interview by M. Mkwate.
129 Interview: Brig. Gertrude Mutasa, *The Sunday Mail*, 11–16 February 2007. Interview by M. Mkwate.
130 Interview: Akwino Aquous Muwoni, aka Texan Chidhakwa, *The Sunday Mail*, 5–11 May 2013. Interview by M. Huni.
131 Interview: Marjorie M. Makaza, Mutare, 17 April 2015.
132 Interview: Akwino Aquous Muwoni, aka Texan Chidhakwa, *The Sunday Mail*, 5–11 May 2013. Interview by M. Huni.
133 Interview: Akwino Aquous Muwoni, aka Texan Chidhakwa, *The Sunday Mail*, 5–11 May 2013. Interview by M. Huni.
134 Report of the Secretary for Health for the year ending 31 December 1977.
135 Interview: Akwino Aquous Muwoni, aka Texan Chidhakwa, *The Sunday Mail*, 5–11 May 2013. Interview by M. Huni.
136 Interview: Akwino Aquous Muwoni, aka Texan Chidhakwa, *The Sunday Mail*, 5–11 May 2013. Interview by M. Huni.
137 Interview: Akwino Aquous Muwoni, aka Texan Chidhakwa, *The Sunday Mail*, 5–11 May 2013. Interview by M. Huni.
138 Interview: Marjorie M. Makaza, Mutare, 17 April 2015.
139 Interview: Akwino Aquous Muwoni, aka Texan Chidhakwa, *The Sunday Mail*, 5–11 May 2013. Interview by M. Huni.
140 Interview: Akwino Aquous Muwoni, aka Texan Chidhakwa, *The Sunday Mail*, 5–11 May 2013. Interview by M. Huni.
141 Interview: Akwino Aquous Muwoni, aka Texan Chidhakwa, *The Sunday Mail*, 5–11 May 2013. Interview by M. Huni.
142 Interview: Marjorie M. Makaza, Mutare, 17 April 2015.
143 Interview: Brig. Felix Muchemwa, *The Sunday Mail*, 17–23 March 2013. Interview by M. Huni.

6

The trajectories of nursing in independent Zimbabwe, 1980–96

In Zimbabwe, just as elsewhere, the end of colonial rule and the coming of independence ushered in a new era. Amongst other things, the new government faced an enormous task in revolutionising the health sector. For this work, the task placed emphasis on transforming the hospital system and, by extension, nurses' working conditions. Besides expanding the health delivery system,[1] the new government took various steps to deracialise and democratise hospitals. The deracialisation and democratisation of hospitals in the first years of independence took two forms. First, the government opened all hospitals to all Zimbabweans, irrespective of race or class. Second, the government continued with the process of Africanising hospital personnel, in particular appointing a greater number of Africans in senior positions in hospitals. The manner in which the first Minister of Health, Dr H. Ushewokunze, implemented the deracialisation and democratisation of hospitals stoked up racial tensions in the new independent nation. Related to nurses, the government made an effort to improve their working conditions. While the government managed to put into motion the deracialisation and democratisation of hospital spaces together with improving working conditions, they still faced numerous challenges in the first decade of independence. As in the colonial period, high numbers of patients and inadequate resources hampered the effective provision of services to the majority.

The problems affecting hospitals and, by extension, nurses in the post-colonial era took a significant turn at the very beginning of the second decade of independence. Two important issues affected nurses' everyday work in hospitals. First, the adoption of austerity measures by the government had a significant impact in the reduction of the health budget as well as investment in public health, with austerity measures eroding the achievements made in the health sector in the first decade of independence. Second, the emergence of HIV/AIDS worsened the situation in hospitals by the mid-1990s. In response to the changing work environment, nurses deployed various coping strategies to ease the burden of working with limited resources and to cushion themselves from the vagaries of the changing economic environment. These strategies included petitions, industrial action and income-generating projects.

The responses elicited controversy as they seemed to indicate a deviation from the traditional notions of nursing and nurses' responsibilities to patients. Nursing is traditionally understood to be based on the concept of practitioners that are satisfied with the duty to care. They are not expected to engage in activities seeking to determine the best way to realise this obligation. For some, the deployment of such a repertoire of coping strategies amounted to a betrayal of their oath to save lives. The adopted coping strategies reflected nurses' deeply held responsibility to patients, commitment to their work and desire to deliver the best care in a tough environment. The strategies, however, created divisions, conflicts and tensions within the nursing fraternity – highlighting what Marks called a 'divided sisterhood'.[2]

Democratising hospitals

At independence, the new government's immediate and major task was to transform the discriminatory and skewed health system. There was an inequitable distribution of health resources in colonial Zimbabwe, and the quality of healthcare differed according to race, social class and region. Infant mortality among white Zimbabweans was around 17 per thousand while in rural areas, where the majority of Africans lived, the rate was as high as 200–300 per thousand.[3] Differences also existed among Africans. Infants born in urban areas had better chances of living through childhood than rural infants. As Samuel T. Agere noted, for every 1,000 babies born in Mufakose, an African suburb in the capital of Harare, twenty-one died in the first year of their birth. In the remote Binga district, infant mortality was 300 for every thousand babies born.[4] Furthermore, a whole range of social inequalities mirrored disparities that existed in the health status of ordinary Zimbabweans. In the capital Harare for example, the government spent twice as much on white patients in comparison to African patients by 1980.[5] Just before independence, the racial breakdown of general hospital beds gave one bed for every 219 Europeans and one bed for every 525 Africans.[6] European hospitals were better equipped with more trained personnel and modern technology than African hospitals. In this regard, the Mugabe government shouldered the responsibility of bridging the massive gap in the provision of health services between races, social classes and regions.

To meet the needs of the people, the government had to address such anomalies. Towards this end, the new government adopted a policy of 'Equity in Health'.[7] Influenced by socialist leanings of the new government and mindful of the injustices of the colonial era, authorities designed the policy to, *inter alia,* deracialise and democratise the provision of health services.[8] The government completed the opening up of hospitals to everyone irrespective of their race, economic status or place of origin; a process that had begun in the late colonial period. In September 1980, the British Broadcasting Corporation reported that hospitals such as Bindura 'took a move to completely abolish the so-called European wards which were in use during colonial days ... the matron of the hospital Mrs Jones, moved ten black patients into the (European) wards, saying it is wrong to have patients overcrowded in other sections of the hospital when there is room in the so-called European wards'.[9] Of course, Bindura was not the only one. Other hospitals followed by completing the deracialisation of clinical spaces after the Ministry of Health had stressed its 'determinations to scrape off all traces of discrimination in the country's medical services structure'.[10] Undeniably, there were significant changes in the healthcare delivery system within the first few years of independence. On a personal level, these changes included free healthcare for those earning less than Z$I50 per month. The free services included 'free in-patient and out-patient treatment, including such things as drugs, dressings and any other diagnostic and other specialist services available in clinics and hospitals run by the government, councils and missions'.[11] Likewise, infant health was the major focus of the Mugabe government. Hence, in 1981 the government initiated an expanded immunisation programme against the six major childhood infectious diseases, and tetanus immunisation of pregnant women. The percentage of children between twelve and twenty-three months immunised in rural Zimbabwe rose from 25 to 42 per cent between 1982 and 1984.[12] The government also started infrastructural developments. These included a vigorous construction and upgrading programme for healthcare facilities. By January 1987, the government had completed 224 rural health centres.[13] In addition, they also earmarked a number of provincial and district hospitals as well as many rural clinics for upgrading. This was a great achievement on the part of the government.

The democratisation of the health system took many forms. While the government was busy on the legislative side, repealing laws such as the Hospital Services Act,[14] the new Minister of Health, Dr Ushewokunze, was waging his own war to transform clinical spaces. Ushewokunze's main goal was to make comprehensive changes to how hospitals conducted their business. It is important to appreciate that the end of the liberation war did not mean an instantaneous change to attitudes and ideas on the part of some sections of the white minority. Others still obstinately held to the racial ideologies and superiority that had always been the hallmark of the colonial era.[15] As many felt, from those in government to ordinary people and across the political spectrum, there was a need for a new war, a war to totally change ideas and attitudes of those (mainly whites) whose intent was to stay in a new Zimbabwe. Ushewokunze was one of the apostles of this new deracialisation process and he used his position as the Minister of Health to proselytise this new gospel. Ushewokunze strongly believed that if the white minority were averse to change, force had to be used or else they had to pack their bags and leave the country. He attacked the colonial mentality 'that hampered the democratisation of institutions'.[16] Ushewokunze noted that 'the forces confronting us in our efforts to end colonial rule and entrenched white supremacy, to create a socialist society, are strong and formidable … The health care system inherited by this government was the creation of a colonial state and, as such, was permeated by the colonial mentality which, as you know, is still the situation today.'[17] Ushewokunze resolved to ensure that African patients were treated with respect, and segregation within hospitals was immediately done away with. As he argued in one of his speeches:

> The transition to genuine black majority rule has not necessarily always been accompanied by a positive or genuine change in racial attitudes that have for decades been entrenched in the provision of health care resources and legislation in this country. Sometimes direct approach and shock tactics are needed to facilitate such change.[18]

Ushewokunze was a man of his word and he strongly believed that his efforts would bear fruit.

Ushewokunze's conduct became the most controversial approach. His conduct received negative press reviews at home and abroad. Three cases come to mind that clearly showed the minister's approach. In July 1980, he visited the Ingutsheni Mental Hospital in Bulawayo. Ushewokunze gave a scathing indictment of the institution, condemning the authorities for their continued dissimilar treatment of patients. At Ingutsheni, 'black patients had horrible food, walked barefoot and were indiscriminately mixed despite the type of mental illnesses'.[19] He reprimanded the authorities for their failure to equitably distribute resources amongst patients. Ushewokunze was not revengeful, Nomsa Makoni argued, rather, he wanted a fair distribution of the limited resources that hospitals received from government. Furthermore, as she argued, he wanted to make sure that 'those who used to oppress us change their attitude and treat us with respect'.[20] At Ingutsheni, he was incensed that with all the help the institution was receiving, racial differences amongst patients were still playing a significant factor in the distribution of the resources. He was enraged that 'the white patients had more facilities than their numbers warranted'.[21] Ushewokunze was determined to put an end to this discrimination. According to Lynette A. Jackson, he managed to do that.[22]

The Minister of Health did not spare other hospitals either as he made it his custom of making impromptu visits to hospitals. It is not clear from the information consulted on the number of hospitals he visited within his first year as the minister. What is clear was that the possibility of unannounced visits caused hospital staff to be always vigilant. Nomsa Makoni remembered that 'there were rumours circulating during the 1980s that the minister visited Harare Hospital and pretended to be a patient, only for nurses to take their time serving him. It is said he gave them a mouthful.'[23] This might have been a rumour as Nomsa Makoni indicated, but Ushewokunze's approach no doubt sent shivers up the spines of nurses of all races. At Gwelo Provincial Hospital, the minister criticised the nursing personnel on unfair patient treatment, made a senior sister cry, and left the nursing staff, black and white alike, very distressed. *The Herald* reported:

> Minister of Health Ushewokunze stormed through Gwelo Hospital yesterday, twice reducing a senior sister to tears and upsetting staff. He peered into linen cupboards, entered almost every closet, chattered to patients, cross-examined nurses and sisters and often appeared angry. This was particularly so when a sister told him that patients drank tea out of old jam and cocoa tins.[24]

Just as at Ingutsheni, Ushewokunze was furious at what he saw as indecorous treatment of patients. He pressed senior nurses not to be afraid to request supplies for the hospital from the government, but also that they must make a tremendous effort in changing their attitude and play their part towards the building of a new Zimbabwe.

The most infamous incident took place at the former all-white hospital, Andrew Fleming (later named Parirenyatwa). The drama was triggered by the unfair treatment of ex-ZANLA combatants by a senior white sister at the hospital.[25] In August 1980, three former combatants were involved in an accident. Injured, they were rushed to Parirenyatwa. Upon arrival, the sister in charge in the casualty ward refused to treat them. The main reason for the refusal was that 'her relative had been killed in war by guerrillas'.[26] The sister in charge left the treatment of the former combatant to African nurses, who reported the incident to hospital authorities.[27] The sister in charge's decision to refuse treating ex-guerrillas was unethical in the sense that nurses are supposed to put the lives of their patients at the forefront. Furthermore, this was an unwise decision on the part of the sister in charge. By refusing to nurse the patient, there is no doubt that she would be branded as one of those ex-Rhodesians still wedded to the past, those who were unwilling to appreciate the winds of change that were blowing across the country. If the sister's behaviour suggested that there were people who were still clinging to the past, hospital administrators did not help either. Their response also suggested that they were still stuck in the past, turning a blind eye to the 'transgression' of a white nurse on black patients. Thus, hospital authorities did not caution or discipline the sister but instead pretended that nothing had happened. When he got wind of the incident, the Minister of Health was furious at the sister and the authorities. He went to the hospital, harangued senior personnel and threatened some of them with immediate dismissal. He also rounded up nurses, gave them a lecture on ethics in nursing and the need to change their attitude, and issued a strong warning that the new government would not tolerate racism within clinical spaces. After that, he showed them a film on the Chimoio massacre.[28] When a white nurse tendered her resignation in the aftermath of the incident, authorities turned it down.

The drama that unfolded at Parirenyatwa Hospital was important as it gives a rare view into examining racial tensions within clinical spaces just after independence, and the tensions and suspicions amongst Zimbabweans in general. The Parirenyatwa Hospital incident became the talk of the town. *The Sunday Mail* editorial implored the Prime Minister to curb Ushewokunze's activities, who 'storm[s] round the country like a rogue elephant, denigrating white members of the medical profession and making the wildest of accusations'.[29] Some members of the white community felt aggrieved. Not only were they disappointed with Ushewokunze's behaviour, they were also angry over what they perceived as the spirit of revenge that was stifling the possibilities of white and blacks working together to build a new Zimbabwe. *The Sunday Mail* was clear, if the minister was allowed to continue with his antics, 'Mr Mugabe's policy of reconciliation [could] stand no chance of success'.[30]

The most vocal of this section of the white community were the representatives of the Republican Front in parliament.[31] They accused the minister of sowing seeds of hatred and propagating mistrust amongst the people. The former Minister of Health in the Ian Smith government, R. Cronje, admonished Ushewokunze for his 'unprofessional' conduct and for bringing the entire medical profession into disrepute. According to Cronje:

> Over the last few months, starting at Ingutsheni Hospital in Bulawayo, then at Gwelo, and culminating in the regrettable meeting that was held at AFH [Andrew Fleming Hospital] in the last weeks, the Minister of Health,

I believe in his conduct and his speeches, and his actions has caused some embarrassment to his office and has given reason for serious concern and insult to the people of the medical profession who with dedication, have followed their calling. I believe what has happened at the AFH harms this country and harms government in several ways. I believe that in hospitals which up to now have built relationships between the staff of all races – as probably a good relationship as there has never been before. It [the minister's conduct] has harmed the relationship between these people. I believe the abuse and criticism and insults which were hurled at the medical and nursing staff at the hospitals, which has not been confirmed, or proved, and in very general terms, has certainly harmed the image of the government, which many other ministers and government as a whole has built up painstakingly over the weeks.[32]

W. D. Walker fully supported Cronje, maintaining that there was 'no need to burden the sick with politics' and if the minister was spoiling for a political fight then 'let us politicians fight if we like to in here [parliament] but never across the beds of the sick patients of the land'.[33] Another Republican Front parliamentarian, R. Cartwright, was more enraged at the minster's behaviour than at the idea behind the minister's actions, which he claimed were stage managed and meant to provoke whites in the country:

The Minister of Health stamps around the country creating unpleasant incident and trouble wherever he goes ... The latest unfortunate incident at AFH (Parirenyatwa) is so typical and so completely unprovoked but nonetheless, carefully stage managed and planned. I have personally visited the Fleming on many occasions both in private and parliamentary capacity and I have always gained the multiracial atmosphere in the hospital. I have seen and visited patients, both black and white being cheerfully and pleasantly cared for by nurses from all communities.[34]

Cartwright maintained that hospitals in Zimbabwe have always been centres of cooperation and good will. The minister, with 'sinister motives', was the one bent on sowing seeds of dissension and ill feeling amongst the staff, blacks and whites. Interestingly, members of the Republican Front deliberately overlooked the fact that hospitals were politicised institutions in Rhodesia. They were quick to forget that they used clinical spaces for political gain, denying African nurses the possibilities of nursing white patients and limiting contact between races in hospitals.

In such a tension-riddled environment, the lines between black and white were starkly drawn. Black legislators fully supported Ushewokunze. The whole purpose of showing the Chimoio massacre video, as G. Chidyausiku argued, was that there were two sides to the war and it was not only whites who suffered from the war, but Africans as well. Chidyausiku emphasised that it was the racialism still prevalent amongst some members of the white community that was a powder keg for instability in the country. Chidyausiku supported the minister's conduct:

> It has also been suggested that the manner in which the minister is handling the whole matter leads to instability. If we allow racialism to continue, then we are creating instability because there was racialism in the past and it led to instability.[35]

More importantly, Chidyausiku reiterated that discrimination was still prevalent in some hospitals:

> These people should be treated with honour. I agree but what is honourable about a person sleeping on the floor in one section of the hospital when there are more than 20 beds empty in the hospital next door and they are not being taken there just because it is being maintained exclusively for the elite [white]. I think it was also reported yesterday that as a result of some of these incidents, hospitals like Bindura are now opening to everybody.[36]

He continued thus:

> If you are black, you do not have to investigate, you just have to go to AFH and you will see the attitude ... I can even recall a few months ago I had to go to AFH for inoculation and you could see the difference of attitude towards blacks and whites by the staff at AFH. Obviously honourable members from across the benches would not be in a position to observe this because they are given preferential treatment.[37]

African MPs categorically sided with Chidyausiku, claiming that discrimination was still rife in former white hospitals. The bone of contention was not the fact that the patients refused attention were former freedom fighters, but that the sister at AFH refused to tend to them on account of their race. This had to be stopped forthwith as many argued.

In his defence, Ushewokunze was unapologetic for his conduct and indicated that he had to do whatever was necessary to democratise and deracialise clinical spaces. It was his responsibility as an appointed minister, to represent the wishes of the majority. In his defence, Ushewokunze said:

> Maybe some members of the house and other interested parties find the concept of direct ministerial involvement in the delivery of health services to the people of Zimbabwe a difficult and most certainly drastic change to the accepted role of the Minister of Health playing the role of a rubber stamp ... To meet health needs I have to utilise a health service structure inherited from the past and potentially hostile to change, a structure that was never designed to meet the needs of the majority of the people whom I represent. This structure must change, or I will not be fulfilling my duties to our people. Therefore, when I am accused of destroying the health services of this country, I should henceforth take it as a compliment. The destruction of discriminatory, archaic and undeniably an unbalanced service would be an act of great service to the people of Zimbabwe. To reconcile oneself to or accept the inherited services as a great achievement on the part of the white man in the past would be tantamount to treason. If the service given is substandard, discriminatory or administered in an irregular manner, the public has every right to voice their feelings. It is my duty to rectify existing inhumanity or malpractices immediately.[38]

The minister received full government support. However, some sections of the white community labelled him a divisive figure bent on destabilising hospitals in the country. Clearly, there is no doubt that the minister's theatrics were unpopular amongst some of the white nurses. Being a transitional period, many were under scrutiny from government officials. White nurses were also under enormous pressure from their African colleagues and patients. Thus, it is highly possible that a significant proportion of white nurses felt uncomfortable in a new environment and the minister's conduct increased the anxiety of life in post-colonial Zimbabwe. African nurses I interviewed had some reservations on the minister's handling of hospital affairs. However, they fully supported the minister, arguing that his conduct was for the greater good of the nation. Doreen Mabika said Ushewokunze's conduct was a bit odd, but that it was necessary:

> As the new Minister of Health in Zimbabwe, he had many responsibilities. He had to turn around the health care system. I think every Zimbabwean who loves their country agreed with his aim. It was his duty to establish and raise the highest possible standards of health care in independent Zimbabwe. He had the duty to warn abusers in the health care sector that it

cannot be tolerated in a democratic non-racial society, so that all nurses and medical staff, irrespective of their race, may know as what the guidelines and boundaries were.[39]

She maintained that it was his responsibility, where necessary, to inform nursing and medical staff of the feelings and experiences and rights of patients. Furthermore, it was his duty to make sure that public expectations in hospitals were met.

In the post-colonial period, hospital desegregation completed the Africanisation of clinical spaces that began in the 1950s and ushered in a new era in hospital relations. Besides repealing The Hospital Service Act in 1981 and Ushewokunze's approach, the new government appointed a number of senior African nurses to influential positions in hospitals. For example, while in 1979 there was only one Chief Nursing Officer, in 1983 the government had increased the number to seven.[40] Chief Nursing Officers were responsible for steering new nursing policies at provincial levels. In addition, they created new posts of Principal Matrons. Principal Matrons worked hand in hand with Chief Nursing Officers at provincial hospitals to make sure that nurses' and patients' needs were met.[41] Nomsa Makoni remembered the changes she saw unfolding in the 1980s, 'Africans took up some of the senior positions after independence. This did not mean that whites were demoted or chased. The president was very reconciliatory and asked them (whites) to stay so that they can help in the development of the country.'[42] Besides promoting African nurses to senior ranks, the government abandoned nursing grades that were based on race. According to Nomsa Makoni,

> We were now equals. It did not matter whether you were white, black, coloured or Indian. The war was fought for equality and that is what transpired in hospitals. As long as you had your qualifications, we were on the same level and received similar treatment and equal salary. And patients were treated the same irrespective of their race.[43]

This was unthinkable during the colonial period. Independence brought other changes to the workplace environment. For nurses, issues surrounding split shifts, night-duty allowances and maternity leave became immediate rallying points. Nelia Ncube reiterated that:

> During the colonial period we could not complain, otherwise one would be fired. But in the post-colonial period, the government was open

minded and requested suggestions on how to improve our working conditions. Because of the nature of our job, the split shift was one of the major concerns. It was terrible for one to go work at 8 am and knock off at 1 pm and then come back at 4 pm and knock off at 8 pm We requested our superiors to change this so that we could have a straight 8 am to 4pm shift and another from 4pm to 8pm shift just like the straight night duty. All these splits were an inconvenience to us when we took into account transport to and from work.[44]

Nurses maintained that the 4:00–8:00 p.m. shift put them in danger as some were mugged at night, and in most cases they experienced transport problems. It must be pointed out that this was not a novel phenomenon. A perusal of newspapers and information from interviews clearly indicates the prevalence of nurses being robbed and experiencing transport problems during the colonial period. However, what changed in the post-colonial period was the social environment that allowed nurses greater space to air their grievances.

The government also introduced night-duty allowances for junior nurses and changed maternity leave policy. During the colonial period there were disparities between junior nurses and senior nurses in terms of night-duty allowances. According to Nelia Ncube, 'a night duty allowance was only paid to those in positions of night superiors, meaning sisters in charge during night duty'.[45] Night-duty allowances were not extended to junior nurses. There is no doubt that this system was discriminatory and the issue surrounding night duty was a bone of contention for many nurses. In 1982, junior nurses pressed the government to immediately change the policy.[46] In December 1983, the government introduced night-shift allowances. The allowance was $4 for nurses and $5 for sisters per night shift. The maximum night allowance per month was $30. No nurse was allowed to earn more than $30 from night allowance. This was to discourage some nurses from demanding perpetual night shifts in order to make more money. Furthermore, the government changed the split shift system by introducing straight shifts and increased uniform allowances.[47]

Nurses also requested that authorities introduce a favourable maternity leave policy. To be sure, in the 1960s, African women working in Civil Service were not offered maternity leave. Once pregnant, they had to resign from the service and reapply after delivery. J. Marere and Mrs Hadebe clearly remembered the predicament they faced as nurses and mothers. J. Marere resigned twice to have two children. According to Mrs Marare,

> During my second pregnancy my husband even suggested that I quit completely. But we needed the money and so I reapplied for my job. The issue of pension was important to every employee because back then people could survive on pensions once they retired. I forfeited all that because I wanted to be a mother.[48]

Mrs Hadebe echoed similar sentiments:

> I resigned four times to have my children and it affected their spacing. The first-born is seven years older than the second, who is five years older than the third who is five years older than the next. The remaining two are spaced from each other by four years.[49]

During the 1960s, many nurses forfeited benefits and pensions once they resigned. While the government amended the policy in the 1970s, it was still unfavourable for working women. Instead of resigning, women would take unpaid maternity leave. This policy was carried over into the first three years of independence and was a source of indignation for many. Labour relations issues were not only a preserve of nurses, but were part of working women's struggles in post-colonial Zimbabwe. Thus, it is important to appreciate that when the government introduced paid maternity leave in 1984, it was extended to all working women in Zimbabwe. It is important to contextualise working women's struggle for maternity leave. The struggle for independence was also based on women's independence. In the immediate post-independence period, issues like the right to full pay, the right to equal treatment, training and opportunities, the right to maternity protection and the right to combine work and domestic responsibilities, were seen as part of women's emancipation.[50] Khan and Jazdowska argued that some of these were superficially addressed. Still the government tried to fulfil some of its obligations to female workers. In 1984, the government passed the Labour Relations Act (1984). This Act made it an offence for an employer to discriminate against any employee or prospective employee on grounds of race, tribe and place of origin, political opinion, colour, creed or sex. The Act also enabled women to take ninety days of maternity leave, earning up to 75 per cent of their salaries.[51] The promulgation of the law was a relief for many.

While it is true to mention that the government tried its best to make sure that their needs were met, nurses still experienced challenges and problems in their daily work. One of the challenges nurses faced was the increased scrutiny of their work by the public. This increased scrutiny and criticism of nurses was partly a result of people's expectations of them and a reflection of the independence euphoria.

> You would hear and sometimes read in the papers allegations that we, nurses at Harare Hospital were not disciplined and we do what we want and we were rough with patients. In fact, these complaints not only pointed fingers at nurses, but also claimed that almost every department, from the administrative desk to assistants and other hospital labourers were guilty of being callous and ill-treated patients seeking medical care.[52]

A complaint of such a nature was published in *Moto*, June 1981. It claimed that patient–nurse relations at the Harare Hospital were virtually non-existent as nurses were rude and cruel:

> The way patients are handled surely makes stories which would make a term in prison look like a holiday in paradise. For as long as I can remember I have witnessed, personally experienced and been told stories of horrifying patient treatment at the hands of black medical personnel. Patients have often dreaded going to government hospitals whether urban or rural, for the simple reason that a visit to these institutions provoked reactions from medical personnel, which seems to suggest the sick person had committed the crime of trespass. No matter how well you tried to behave yourself, you could never hope to escape being scolded. As it was impossible to find a reasonable explanation for these people's outbursts, the only logical conclusion most people come to was that it must have been considered a crime to fall sick.[53]

One would assume from the above report in *Moto* magazine that within a year of independence, nurses had turned Harare Hospital into the most inhospitable and uncharitable place. *Moto* was not the only culprit in its negative portrayal of nurses, government newspapers also carried what they claimed to be cases of ill treatment of patients in hospitals, suggesting that nurses in post-colonial Zimbabwe had become callous, cruel and were more interested in lining their pockets than taking care of the sick. In 1983, for example, *The Sunday Mail* claimed that nursing was replete with undedicated young women: 'Today's nurses are different from yesterdays' in that they are not willing to get pittance as a reward after a month's work. Most are taking nursing as a stepping stone into the private sector.'[54] There were many nurses who were moving to the private sector as it paid better than the public sector. However, to suggest that nurses had all but abandoned their duty was being mendacious. Without trying to defend some nurses who might have been callous, many nurses continued doing their best in offering services to the new nation. Such complaints about nurses can be traced to the high expectations of service in the aftermath of independence. Independence ushered in a crisis of high expectation that was felt in all parts of Zimbabwean society and hospitals were not spared. Nurses, on their part, had their own expectations that their situation and working conditions would drastically change for the better within clinical spaces. But they also had to shoulder the burden of patients' expectations. Nomsa Makoni summed the issue up well when she said, 'everyone who came to receive treatment at the hospital expected to be treated like royalty because we were now independent. Thus, if nurses failed to meet their expectation, they labelled them cruel, lazy and so forth.'[55]

An examination of health reforms in the 1980s indicates that, although there were impressive gains for nurses and patients alike, there were a number of problems in the health sector that needed government attention by the end of the decade. For example, there was a continued disparity in wealth and income between Zimbabwean elites (black and white) and the majority continued to 'generate differences in the type and extent of morbidity in different social classes in Zimbabwe'.[56] During the colonial period, race was the main determining factor in the provision of services; by the end of the 1980s, class differences perpetuated unequal access to health resources. In terms of hospitals and nurses' work, the former 'white only' hospitals like Parirenyatwa Hospital and United Bulawayo Hospital continued to enjoy better facilities and smaller workloads than their sister hospitals, Harare and Mpilo. By the end of the 1980s, Harare and Mpilo remained the 'poorer sisters'.[57] For example, the input cost for patient care in 1988 was $38.67 for Harare and $92.76 for Parirenyatwa.[58] By the end of the 1980s, lack of adequate resources at former African-only hospitals hampered the effective provision of services to the majority.

Austerity measures and HIV/AIDS

The situation took a major downturn with the adoption of austerity measures in Zimbabwe, known as the Economic Structural Adjustment Programme (ESAP), coupled with the pressures brought by the resurgence of TB and the emergence of HIV/AIDS. In 1990, Zimbabwe adopted ESAP in response to increasing problems affecting the economy. The government started implementing the programme in 1991. As with other programmes implemented in parts of Africa, central to ESAP was the restructuring of the economy through 'demand management, currency devaluation, trade liberalization, and elimination of price control'.[59] ESAP also required the government to increase interest rates to their natural level to discourage capital flight, the reduction of the budget deficit, and the removal of government subsidies on goods and services.[60] The Zimbabwean government was also compelled to reduce its spending on public health. As a result, the real per capita expenditure on health in Zimbabwe dropped by 33.8 per cent within three years of the implementation of ESAP.[61]

The introduction of ESAP gradually eroded the country's health success. The Zimbabwe government reduced its health budget and transferred costs to the consumer as part of the conditions to receive funding.[62] The devaluation of the Zimbabwe dollar and the rise in inflation aggravated the situation. By 1992, inflation and devaluation had, in real terms, reduced the health budget by 20 per cent.[63] The impact was immediate. Personal interviews with practising health professionals reveal that they could see the impending disaster within the programme's first two years.[64] Government officials pointed out in 1992 that the situation had deteriorated at an alarming rate. The Minister of Health and Child Welfare, Timothy Stamps, publicly acknowledged that ESAP had become the number one threat to public health, whilst his deputy, Tsungirirayi Hungwe, requested that the country's health delivery system be declared a 'national disaster "in order to avoid a" complete breakdown in health services'.[65] Such a rare acknowledgement of government's failure to maintain standards indicated the enormity of the problems that affected the public health sector within a space of two years after ESAP implementation.

As might have been expected, the deterioration of working conditions matched the decline in public health investment. Viola

Moyo recalled how, by 1992, she began to notice changes at her workplace, whilst Laiza Shumba remembered that by 1993, 'it was becoming clear that hospitals were becoming transit points to graves'.[66] This did not mean that the majority of patients in hospitals at this time were necessarily terminally ill, rather Laiza Shumba's observation pointed to the changing conditions in hospitals as gravely detrimental to patient health. Reductions in investment meant that administrators had to direct resources towards what they considered as the most essential of services and departments. It also meant less investment in repairs and the replacement of old and obsolete hospital equipment. Interviews confirmed the difficulties that nursing staff faced in their attempts to serve patients' needs under these circumstances. Claris Bere recalled that for much of 1993, the ultrasound scan and cardiotocography machines, essential for foetal monitoring, were out of order. The hospital had problems in fixing the machines and lacked the financial capacity to replace them. The nurses, therefore, encountered enormous challenges as they tried to diagnose and deal with complications amongst maternity patients.[67] Other hospitals had their own share of problems. For example, in 1994 only one of the five X-ray machines at Parirenyatwa Hospital was operational and other hospital equipment was frequently inoperative.[68] At times nurses had to wait for days to obtain test results and sometimes requested patients 'to go to private service providers to get scans, X-rays, and other tests done'.[69] The use of private service providers resulted in the marginalisation of a significant proportion of patients, since the less privileged constituted the larger majority of patients who attended public hospitals, who in turn suffered most from a lack of services.

By 1994, other organizations were starting to criticise the conditions that existed in the country's various hospitals. The nurses' organisation, Zimbabwe Nurses Association (ZINA), urged the government to improve the situation within hospitals.[70] ZINA president, Clara Nondo, publicly complained about government's failure to maintain standards and improve working conditions for nurses. Her interview with the labour-based newspaper, *The Worker*, documented her frustrations over the state of affairs in hospitals as noted in the statement that:

> Sometimes we have to watch helpless patients dying because they [hospitals] lacked necessary drugs or equipment to treat them. There is so much frustration that some [nurses] were leaving the country to seek greener pastures.[71]

The shortages and the resultant frustrations to the nursing personnel were vividly chronicled by Flora Matondo in her interview responses outlining the problems faced by nurses during the mid-1990s:

> How would you expect to take care of the sick with almost nothing? Medication was scarce, working utensils were getting antiquated and not being replaced. Some machines were not being serviced. It was tough for us just as it is still today. This did not mean there were no options for us. Some left the country and some went into the private sector. Some of us remained put, hoping that the situation would get better but it did not. Moreover, for the love of the job, the commitment to our patients, we persisted. Endurance was critical. One would be so overwhelmed with work that at times you just do what you can.[72]

The condition continued to deteriorate to the extent that by 1996, the hospital system was in a state of paralysis. An examination of non-nursing services, such as catering amenities, illuminates this point. Information from interviews and reports from newspapers showed that impecunious hospitals were being compelled to scale down the provision of food to patients during the 1995–96 period.[73] There were no reported cases of patient starvation, but the relative shortage of food at Harare Hospital, for example, forced the administration to recommend that relatives bring supplementary sustenance for patients. The patients who suffered most under these conditions were those whose close relatives lived outside Harare. One patient complained that:

> The situation here is horrible. Some of us do not have close relatives who can bring us food. What are we to survive on? We are paying tax and we think it is the responsibility of the government to provide that service [providing food].[74]

Thus, various problems affected the provision of medical care in the Zimbabwe of the early 1990s. Nevertheless, the hospitals continued to function as if everything was normal, which bears testimony to nurses' resilience, determination and dedication to their work.

At this time, the government was also confronted by another major problem: the HIV/AIDS pandemic. In 1994 the cumulative number of HIV/AIDS cases since 1987 was at a total of 38,552.[75] As shown in Table 6.1, the number of HIV/AIDS cases increased by 16 per cent between 1993 and 1994, 166 per cent between 1990 and 1994, and 8,847 per cent between 1987 and 1994.

The data used to compile the table was collected mainly from government and mission hospitals. It does not include patients who

Table 6.1 Total number of HIV/AIDS cases by year (national)

Year	Number of cases
1987	119
1988	202
1989	1,311
1990	4,000
1991	4,362
1992	4,557
1993	9,174
1994	10,647

Source: Report of the Secretary for Health and Child Welfare for the year ending 31 December 1994

visited other health institutions for treatment. Nonetheless, HIV/AIDS brought significant changes to the disease environment in hospitals during the 1990s. According to Sunanda Ray and Farai Madzimbamuto, Zimbabwe was one of the earliest countries to start screening blood donors for HIV when the test became commercially available in 1985 after first cases were reported.[76] Furthermore, an excellent volunteer-based system led by the National Blood Donation and Transfusion Service assisted in containing the spread of the virus to clinical spaces.[77] However, a culture of secrecy slowed the implementation of HIV/AIDS education programmes for healthcare workers, as suggested by one informant, Doreen Mabika, here:

> During the late 1980s, we knew that there was this new disease that had a potential of significantly changing occupational health matters with the hospital workforce and altering the relations between hospital workers and patients. But very little was done in hospitals as government's main concern was the curative aspect rather than preventative measures. We were to reap the rewards of government's procrastination in the following decade.[78]

As a result, the limited and haphazard government intervention during the late 1980s left many nurses unprepared for what was witnessed in the hospital sector in the 1990s. The relative absence of information about the disease in the early 1990s and the unavailability of antiretroviral drugs such as PEP (post-exposure prophylaxis) that are crucial immediately after exposure, and the general culture of not immediately reporting blood borne pathogen exposure, left many health care workers precariously exposed to the virus.[79]

However, the immediate impact came from the sharp increase in patients with opportunist infections. By 1994, the nurse to patient ratio had increased from 1:5 to 1:35 within a space of three years.[80] The increase, according to the Health Secretary, Sikosana, resulted from 'high numbers of terminally ill largely due to the HIV/AIDS pandemic'.[81] The nurses interviewed during the study complained of the inevitable increased workload due to the coincidental rise in AIDS sufferers in hospitals at a time when hospitals were facing severe shortages in medication and equipment. Jane Mushando pointed out that:

> AIDS caused many problems for us healthcare workers. The disease made our work more difficult than any other time I can remember. When I entered the profession in the 1970s, the disease environment was entirely different from what we have these days. Children, teenagers, young men, women, and even the elders have been victims of the diseases. Hospitals were always full with terminally ill patients. This was the time the government was not doing much in terms of providing a healthy working environment … To make matters worse, hospitals had problems in acquiring protective clothing. Gloves were becoming scarce and imagine having to work without gloves at times.[82]

Jane Mushando's remarks underscored the challenges faced by nurses during the 1990s owing to both the changing disease environment and government-introduced austerity measures. Dr P. L. N. Sikosana, Secretary for Health and Child Welfare, captured what was taking place within hospitals in this way: 'Staff morale continued to fall with the real value of staff salaries deteriorating relative to the cost of living. The sharp increase in the number of chronically ill patients further increased the unbearable pressure on hospital services.'[83] There is no doubt that the AIDS epidemic put nurses under enormous pressure.[84]

'We had to act': Nurses' coping strategies

The appalling hospital conditions compelled some nurses to leave for greener pastures. The Director of Nursing estimated that, by 1997, Zimbabwe had lost close to 1,300 nurses and doctors because of

ESAP and the problems affecting the health sector at the time.[85] The majority, however, remained and faced the obstacles and challenges that were making it tough to provide satisfactory care to patients. The remaining nurses confronted the challenges in various ways, with some nurses going to the extent of buying their own gloves in order to deal with the widespread glove shortage.[86] Nurses, who had to face their patients in the context characterised by reduced investments in health care and drug shortages, also became innovative in an attempt to deal with the shortage of medication. L. A. Bijlmakers. M. T. Bassett and D. M. Sanders noted that patients who were instructed to purchase drugs at private pharmacies would exert pressure on nurses to provide them with medication from the hospital dispensary.[87] As a result, nurses referred patients to clinics or hospitals where the required drugs were available.[88] Furthermore, nurses resorted to second or third line medication to circumvent the drug shortages.[89] This left nurses less than satisfied as they began to view the economic situation as being responsible for making their work tough.

Nurses also became stricter on admissions in order to deal with the surge in patient numbers. Within Zimbabwe's hospital structure, referral hospitals dealt with severe cases that nurses at clinics and district hospitals would have found difficult to treat. During the colonial period, hospital administrators had tried to regulate the number of patients who visited referral hospitals, especially those suffering from minor injuries that could be treated at clinics.[90] However, the post-colonial era witnessed urban hospitals, such as Harare Hospital, becoming less strict as they began to allow non-referral patients. This trend, however, started to change in the 1990s. Claris Bere recollected that:

> When we realised that we are having many people, we encouraged them to visit clinics in their areas first instead of coming straight to hospitals. Of course, we did not turn them away, but we believed that our efforts were meant at reducing our work.[91]

Jane Mushando, in her work at the Mutare General Hospital, also observed a similar trend. Furthermore, she insisted that they encouraged relatives to do their part, especially in taking care of terminally ill patients:

> Because we would be having shortages of staff and there were times when food was scarce, we would weigh the condition of a patient if we realise

that this patient would not survive, we would tell the relatives to take them home and take care of them at home. Of course, they came for check-ups but this had two advantages. We made space for other patients and reduced our workload.[92]

It is hard to measure the success of these coping strategies because of the high turnover of patients in hospitals. However, nurses themselves maintained that the effort went a long way in alleviating the challenges that they had been facing. Yet this sense of doing something about an untenable situation did not play out well in public. The public perceived the strategy as an abandonment of their responsibilities. Statements from the public criticised the quality of service as noted in the complaint that: 'They [nurses] do not want to be in direct contact with patients. All they like is to be proud and to look smart (clean) outside, but they are dirty inside.'[93] This offers clear insight into the general public's feelings about nurses' conduct during the time under discussion.

As was the case with other workers, the decline in real wages compelled a significant number of nurses to seek alternative means to supplement their salaries. Mlambo noted that the early 1990s witnessed the beginning of a trend where wages lagged behind inflation rates. For instance, salary levels for most working people were below the 45 per cent increase in the cost of living in 1993, which resulted in a 35 per cent decline in real wages, and by 1995, average wages had risen by only 45 per cent whilst average prices had doubled during the 1992/93–95 period.[94] The decline in real wages, which also meant the gradual slip of the nursing profession from the traditional middle class,[95] compelled nurses to look for alternative ways to augment their salaries and maintain their households.[96]

The popular and immediate strategy was the implementation of the 'round system/society', a money-saving club commonly known as 'stokvels' in some parts of southern Africa.[97] This was neither new nor exceptional at the time, as it represented a common system in use, especially among women in the informal sector. The clubs were voluntary, based on trust, and did not involve anyone outside the immediate work environment as they were work-related associations. This was necessary to avoid disputes and the numbers were kept to a minimum in order to reduce one's waiting period to access the funds.

The adoption of ESAP resulted in a rise in cross-border trading as a major livelihood survival strategy for many Zimbabweans. Traders travelled mainly to South Africa, Botswana and Zambia to purchase commodities for resale in Zimbabwe. Scholars on cross-border trading agree that such trading became prevalent in the 1990s. The analysis, however, tends to associate cross-border trade with informally employed women.[98] A minority of formally employed women also took up such activities. However, cross-border trading was never easy. It was fraught with challenges such as having one's goods confiscated or stolen. In addition, Estella Dhlamini pointed out that nurses hardly mentioned their profession to other traders while on trading trips in fear of antagonism or muted derision:

> Cross-border trading used to be mainly for *vapostori* (members of the various independent African churches) then it quickly became fashionable amongst women who were formally employed. It was a way of contributing something to the family in the wake of increased tightening of resources. We, however, did not even think that we would one day be involved in such an activity. As a gainfully employed woman, I had a good source of income. However, when the situation worsened, I had no choice but to engage in it as well. In addition, because we were considered privileged, one would not even dare tell other women that you are a nurse. They would laugh at you and say, aaah! Now nurses are nothing but just ordinary people. We are now the same as they are not that special as they used to portray themselves. Therefore, I dared never to mention I was a nurse.[99]

A smiling Estella Dhlamini indicated that she only became comfortable on her second journey. Even when this was the case, nurses had other challenges that were different from other women, for nurses' border-crossing activities were dictated by their work schedules and they could only go out when they were either off duty or during their leave days.

Cross-border trading and, at times, moonlighting in the private sector, impacted negatively on nurses' performance at work. According to Estella Dhlamini:

> Non-nursing activities meant to raise extra cash affected our work in a number of ways. We will come to work mostly tired and we had to endure long working hours and sometimes night duties. Imagine that you had to

go to South Africa or Botswana to buy commodities for resale. It is time consuming and the hassles at the border leave many frustrated. When you come back, you do not have enough time to rest and an absent minded and distracted nurse is not a good nurse. Sometimes you are worried about the merchandise you had to sell since they will be competing with other cross-border traders. That is not good for the patients, and neither will it be of benefit to us as nurses.[100]

A 1993 study expressed similar sentiments. The nurses who were interviewed felt that activities such as moonlighting affected their work and relations with patients in a negative way. One informant noted that:

One used to worry if they made a mistake. You would have many sleepless nights. Now you cannot be bothered. In fact, before ESAP, nurses discussed medicine. Now all they talk about is best ways to deal. Instead of giving health education to patients, you find a nurse busy asking a patient where this or that can be procured.[101]

There can be little doubt that these activities affected the quality of nursing services to patients.

'Mercenaries who fight for money': The August and October–December strikes of 1996

Nurses also resorted to direct confrontation as exemplified by the 1996 strikes. The industrial action became controversial and developed into a tension-filled strike characterised by mixed feelings amongst nurses, which brought to the surface the often hidden militant side within the nursing sorority.[102] In the process, nurses unsettled the Nightingale pledge of suffering for humanity and that of personal satisfaction without much compensation. The strikes, as in other parts of the world, were partly aimed at criticising the policy and ideology that emphasised the service nature of the profession. For example, decades earlier, the USA perceived collective bargaining and unionisation amongst some nurses as a challenge to 'the traditional ideology of service' and indicative of the nurses' rejection of the 'pious exhortations about professional duty'.[103] Similarly, the collective action in Zimbabwe was both a critique and rejection of the idea that nurses must continue serving even in difficult conditions and without proper acknowledgement or adequate remuneration.

Nurses proved to be resilient, vocal and the most visible of the entire Zimbabwean civil service during the August strike. They came out as more committed to their cause and had greater confidence in their potential to change their situation. According to Estella Dhlamini:

> We could not just work under poor conditions and for almost free ... At the time, this was a wound that was destroying the nursing profession. By not negotiating in good faith, the government was just trying to paper over the wound with a Band-Aid. We said no, the government must commit itself to improve our situation.[104]

It is not surprising that the government's failure to show immediate commitment to the civil servants' demands resulted in the nurses' joining together with junior doctors and going on strike again on 21 October 1996. This further strike was triggered by the government's failure to negotiate honestly with healthcare workers. The government seemed less committed to meet conditions set by nurses to the extent that it postponed consultations with nurses' representatives three times in September and was reneging on its promises to improve the working environment in hospitals.

An anatomy of the course the strike took unsettled the often-perceived homogeneity within the nursing sorority and exposed what Shula Marks explained as a 'divided sisterhood'.[105] It was mainly junior nurses who went on strike in October. While on one level the strike showed the organisational capacity of junior nurses, on the other level it exposed the gulf between the strikers and their seniors. Such a situation meant that bigger referral hospitals in urban areas remained partially functional, with nursing orderlies and student nurses helping senior nurses, while the smaller hospitals, more dependent on a junior nursing establishment, were left vulnerable.

ZINA had failed to assess the situation. ZINA was the only public service association that did not support the strike in August on the grounds that the strike was politically motivated.[106] Ironically, its members came to be the most militant and committed to using the strike route.[107] Again in October, ZINA distanced itself from the strike as it did not overtly sympathise with the striking nurses. Their failure to sanction and subsequently support the strike led to a showdown with nurses, especially when they tried to intervene. ZINA president, Clara Nondo, addressed the striking nurses on 21 October in an attempt to urge them to rethink their position and convince them to return to work whilst they entered into new negotiations with the government.[108] The speech was met with interjections and interpolations, jeering and name-calling, thus indicating the divisions that existed amongst nurses and how nursing leadership had become out of touch with its constituency. Nurses further went on to appropriate the everyday revolutionary discourse used by the ruling party and the government, to accuse the association of 'selling out' their cause to the government.[109] Such interjections and the appropriation of political discourses showed the junior nurses' spirit of defiance and independence from the leadership, which in the process exposed a high level of militancy within the nursing sector.

The government's initial response displayed its arrogance towards nurses and junior doctors. No one illustrated such conceit better than the then acting Minister of Labour and Social Welfare, Nathan Shamuyarira, who claimed that the reasons for the strike 'were unknown and the move unreasonable'.[110] Hospital administrators and other senior medical personnel at hospitals followed suit and went on to maintain that the situation was under control. Events on the ground, however, revealed a different and disturbing scenario, for the impending disaster and chaos were beginning to unfold at hospitals in metropolitan Harare by the second day of the strike. The withdrawal of labour was so overwhelming that Parirenyatwa and Harare hospitals closed a number of wards, in spite of the fact that some senior nurses, student nurses and medical orderlies had not joined the strike.[111] The third day witnessed a discontinuation of all non-emergency units at Parirenyatwa, while obstetrics and gynaecology cases were transferred to Harare Hospital where more room was available.[112] The presence of senior nurses and student nurses at Harare Hospital made the performance of emergency operations possible. However, fear of intimidation from other nurses made their work difficult. According to Veronica Sibanda: 'I did not join because I felt that I had to continue with my work. This does not mean I did not sympathise with junior nurses, I did. I felt that we could not close the hospital since we had emergency cases that needed our immediate attention.'[113] Furthermore, senior nurses who did not join the strike were working in civilian clothing for fear of being targeted and victimised by striking nurses.[114] It was reported by the end of the week that only the casualty department seemed to be operating normally at Harare Hospital whilst the rest of the wards were nearly empty.[115]

The strike affected the whole country in different ways. It had spread to Bulawayo and Mutare within a period of three days. The situation at Marondera Hospital was characterised by the presence of a small number of senior nurses that were attending to emergency and maternity cases, with a similar situation prevailing at Chinhoyi Hospital while the state of affairs at Bindura Hospital was described as 'bad'.[116] The 'bad' situation at Chinhoyi was clearly shown as severe in the way that all patients who were admitted were placed in one ward, regardless of their sex and age, due to the staff shortage.[117] In addition, *The Herald* reported after a few weeks into the strike that:

> Both Harare and Parirenyatwa continue to attend to emergency cases only and on Tuesday night, Parirenyatwa admitted 14 critically ill patients, a slightly higher number since the strike started. The hospital has however closed 17 wards and at Harare 13 wards were closed yesterday while 13 others are partially open to accommodate emergency cases. The neo-natal intensive care unit was totally closed.[118]

Thus, it became apparent by 21 November, a month into the strike, that chaos had become the order of the day at most hospitals in the country.

The government responded to the strike in various ways after realising that the situation had become unsustainable. The state, using a divide and rule tactic, reached a separate agreement with junior doctors. The assumption was that the junior doctors' return to work would also trigger the nurses' return. There had been a justifiable belief, within official circles, that nurses were being used by junior doctors and hence negotiating with junior doctors would be akin to the proverbial killing of two birds with one stone. This perception is clearly illustrated in President Mugabe's claim at an international conference in Rome that the strike was directionless and 'the nurses seem to have been commandeered into striking by misguided junior doctors'.[119] Mugabe's remarks are important, for, although they were not an official government statement, they nevertheless reveal the government's inner view regarding the nurses and the strike. Female nurses were considered to be timid, weak and dependent on junior doctors. In other words, nursing was perceived as a handmaid to medicine.[120]

Nurses, however, were not deterred by such accusations. They refused to capitulate and went on to show that they were independent actors who had enough capacity to mobilise and sustain the industrial action on their own. Furthermore, the junior doctors' resumption of practice ironically went on to show that the doctors depended on nurses and not the other way round. No one expressed this better than Tendai Jiah, the representative of the junior doctors, who stated in his admission that, 'we (doctors) have returned to work, yes but we are not working, we are just here in the building and I don't know if it's working'.[121] Another doctor echoed similar sentiments in the statement that, 'we cannot be expected to work without nurses. They are an essential part of our duties.'[122] These statements, therefore, locate nurses at the centre of the hospital matrix. The interviewees maintained that nurses were not just mere helpers to doctors, or the physician's hand, but were pivotal in the hospital system. In addition, there was a low level functioning of health service delivery at the country's major hospitals as the junior doctors literally milled around owing to the absence of nurses. *The Herald* noted that:

> A long queue formed at the casualty and another winding queue formed at the dispensary as most patients, who under normal circumstances would be admitted were given medication to take home. Parirenyatwa Hospital remained chaotic with reports that the hospital was sending some of its patients to Harare Hospital.[123]

It must be underscored that, Harare Hospital, which was supposedly open, was not fully functional, as a significant number of wards remained closed. In fact, most wards at national hospitals across the country remained closed as nurses refused to budge to the government's call that they stop striking and return to work.

The government later realised that the nurses' strike was well organised and they were gaining public sympathy, and as such introduced a new strategy to undermine the impact of the labour activism. The state started using its apparatus to control public spaces, especially those spaces where nurses gathered to spread information and compare tactics. To this end, the police sealed off two public spaces that were used by nurses as their rendezvous – Africa Unity Square and Harare Gardens.[124] In addition, the police camped at hospital grounds to stop anyone from a list of 2,000 nurses and 232 junior doctors who went on strike from entering the hospital premises in an attempt to prevent the intimidation of nurses who had refused to join the strike.[125] The Deputy Commissioner of Police, Tandabantu Godwin Matanga, clearly stated the police strategy when he pointed out that, 'Police have moved into hospitals following reports of intimidation received recently, during which those who had volunteered were being forced to leave their premises ... such action would not be tolerated and any people [nurses] found intimidating others into joining the strike will be charged for contravening LOMA.'[126] The government also turned to the media, insisting on a media blackout on the nurses' strike and anything related to the strike. However, the government's efforts at information management proved ineffective as nurses used other communication channels, especially telephones. In addition, the weekly private media continued to cover the strike.

The government threatened striking nurses with dismissal. It also declared that the dismissed would be replaced with expatriate workers. Ironically, the authorities failed to realise that it was going to be expensive to hire expatriate workers and that it would most likely hire the very same people who had left the country for greener pastures. Nevertheless, the nurses refused to be cowed into submission, resulting in the government firing all striking workers during the fourth week. Those willing to come back to work had to reapply within a month and had to forfeit their wages for the time they were on strike.[127] The government's decision to fire all striking nurses instead raised their profile as a group that was being sacrificed at the altar of political expediency and in the process attracted many sympathisers to the nurses' cause. Even members of parliament, who usually sided with the government, criticised the state's approach. Mavis Chidzonga's contribution to the parliamentary motion on civil servants condemned some of her colleagues' insensitivity to nurses and patients because:

> They [some government officials] do not have to go Harare Hospital. They fly out and they are not treated at Parirenyatwa Hospital and they are not even treated at Avenues [one of the private hospitals in Harare] as they can afford to go overseas. Their children go overseas. Their relations are overseas. When they have a broken arm or a sore ear they fly out. So our

problem is that those who are concerned with nurses' issues and junior doctors' issues should really ask the government to negotiate with them so that service is provided for us who cannot afford to fly out.[128]

Margaret Dongo, one of the few oppositional members of parliament at the time, emphasised the rights of nurses as workers:

> These are civil servants and it is not a crime to be a civil servant because they have rights as well. These people are not buying bread from different shops and they do not get special discounts and also they are facing difficulties faced by any other individuals who have been affected by the cost of living. So, yes they are essential services but what are not essential services?[129]

Chidzonga, Dongo and other parliamentarians were, in essence, advocating the rights of nurses as workers. What incensed many was the idea that fired nurses were expected to reapply and be treated as first-time applicants. Richard Shambambeva-Nyandoro exposed the problem behind the thinking in his contribution that:

> Some have been in the health system for 10, 15 to 20 years. How can a person who has been employed for twenty years be told that they were starting from a low grade like someone who has just come to look for employment? We have talked to some nurses in our constituencies. That is where the seriousness of the issue is.[130]

It was beyond any reasonable doubt that the proposal was unfair to nurses. Furthermore, the reality that they had to apply on an individual basis meant that there were strong possibilities of victimisation.

Other organisations such as ZimRights and the main labour movement, the Zimbabwe Congress of Trade Unions (ZCTU), also supported the striking nurses.[131] This move supports Richard Sanders' suggestion that the crisis within the labour sector in the 1990s brought disparate labour movements together.[132] In fact, the ZCTU organised a mass protest supporting the striking nurses and junior doctors. The police tear-gassed the marchers, a condition that elicited further ZCTU response in which they organised a two-day mass stay-away seeking to force the government to restore the operational capacity of hospitals. The ZCTU also urged the government to respect the workers' right to express themselves through demonstration.[133] The two-day mass stay-away was a flop. However, it showed the potential of worker solidarity that crossed narrow professional lines. This camaraderie was to be fully exploited by the ZCTU in the coming years.

Interestingly, the public, which initially sympathised with nurses, began to shift its support owing to the continued closure of hospitals. The longer nurses remained on strike, the more the tide of public sympathy shifted away from them. Particularly important is that public responses exposed the complexities of the nursing profession, especially the nature of work, tensions over patient rights and the perception that nurses have to serve the patient irrespective of the working conditions. As a result, the anti-strike propaganda campaigners took advantage of the public's fatigue with the strike and began whipping public sentiments against nurses by making it a moral issue. An editorial in *The Sunday Mail* exposed this shift in attitude:

> The whole issue has now assumed a moral dimension and public sympathy which was once with the striking nurses (and doctors) is turning away from them. Their attitude is increasingly being seen as not compatible with the calling and ethics of their profession. The cold-heartedness of leaving a patient dying while clamouring for more payment is not consistent with the image set by Nightingale ... the nursing profession is more of a calling than anything and demands dedication that money cannot buy. Questions are being asked as to what kinds of relationship the nurses (and doctors) are establishing with their patients and government.[134]

The message, which sought to blackmail nurses emotionally, was that nurses must listen to their conscience and end the strike. It also stated that the nurses had to put their patients first and continue the negotiations while at work.[135] This appeal to the nurses' conscience enabled the anti-strikers to remove the burden and patient responsibility from authorities and place it squarely on the shoulders of the nurses. Moreover, another editorial in *The Herald* accused workers of being both too militant in their demands and embarking on 'silly' strikes at the expense of patients. The editorial stated:

> Doctors and nurses know that they can make their point more effectively than all other professions. They have our lives in their hands. Last time they went on strike many lives were lost ... If Air Zimbabwe engineers can strike and ground aircraft and the corporation lose millions of dollars and the good of the passengers, why should doctors not put down their tools as

well? That kind of thinking is frightening to say the least. More also when lives being bargained with are those of the poor who have nowhere else to go. Whether or not the doctors and nurses' grievances are genuine and whatever they are, they are betraying the oath to save lives. They cannot, at whim, just withdraw their labour. There are ethical matters they should consider. Now they have blood on their hands. How do people forgive them? How can people trust them? … If anyone is enjoying the show, they have not seen the escalating body count.[136]

Morality, duty and respect for patient rights became the final rallying point for those opposed to the strike. Nurses' action had ceased being a problem of working conditions and was being constructed as a breach of medical ethics as patient bodies became a new terrain of struggle.

The issues revolving around life, well-being and death of patients became the immediate rallying point during this strike period. An emphasis on patients' rights to medical care over nurses' rights as workers became an easy route for both the authorities and anti-strike constituency. A letter from one Chikwapuro read:

> Nurses are under oath to save life and nowhere does the oath give an exception that when they want an increase in salaries they should disregard the oath and allow people to die. Our nurses and junior doctors have become mercenaries who fight for money and disregard human life. They have damaged the image of the nurse and the profession as a whole. Their profession, which was considered noble, now consists of people who could be called witches who do not care about the death of the loved ones … It is important that the government should never compromise … We do not need nurses of this nature who are anti-nursing and have no sense of responsibility[137]

Categories such as witches, mercenaries and sell-outs have long historical roots in Zimbabwe's everyday discourse. Witches and witchcraft are associated with harming instead of healing, and they conjure up death rather than maintain life. Thus, the deployment of such categories on nurses and linking the continuation of the industrial strike with the mounting body count in hospitals, defined the nurses as having forfeited their duty to heal and preserve life and transformed them into agents of grief and death. Likewise, the use of the category of mercenary has been employed in Zimbabwe's social, political and cultural discourses to label people who are not considered worthy or patriotic enough. The category was mainly used during the liberation struggle and the 1980s civil war, yet it was now being deployed by the government on civilians whom they thought were opposed to their regime. In essence, the deployment of such categories was aimed at denying nurses their civic right to industrial action and marginalising their concerns.

The nurses that I interviewed described the deployment of such categories and the negative attention they received as unfair and unjustified. Such categories, as informants maintained, undervalued their contribution to the nation's well-being.[138] A letter to *The Sunday Mail* by an unnamed nurse illustrates these sentiments concisely:

> Our not taking industrial action in the past has been misconstrued to mean nurses are angels who are expected to give and take nothing in return … Nursing is a profession and requires salaries commensurate with the work but to try and convince policy makers that nurses' salaries are not adequate is met with hostility and seen as being unpatriotic. At present government regards nurses as allied staff that provide services to professionals such as doctors and it is unclear if this is the reason government has taken long to deal with nurses' demands … For how long shall patients continue to suffer, with the government taking its time to solve the nurses and other health personnel's problems?[139]

This extract documents the nurses' reiteration that the main reason for the strike was government's failure to view them as professionals who deserve better working conditions and a salary that is proportionate with their input.[140] It is not surprising, therefore, that the longer the industrial action took, the more vocal the public became against nurses. Ultimately, this resulted in nurses becoming more disillusioned. The government also refused to negotiate with laid off nurses and increased its witch-hunt against the leaders of the strike. As a result, it became apparent to the striking nurses that they were fighting a losing battle. One cannot pin down an exact date when the strike ended as it was never called off. Rather, nurses began to trek back to work on an individual basis, with the government promising that they would not victimise them. Some of the nurses, however, felt aggrieved and left the profession, while others left the country for greener pastures. In total, the government struck off 278 nurses from the register.[141]

Conclusion

In 1980, the white community in Salisbury (Harare) severely criticised Dr H. S. M. Ushewokunze, the new Minister of Health in Zimbabwe, for reprimanding white nurses at Andrew Fleming (Parirenyatwa) Hospital. The white community saw the admonishment as going against the spirit of reconciliation and bordering on vengefulness. Ushewokunze, however, envisioned it differently.

To him, it was part of the deracialisation of hospital spaces in post-colonial Zimbabwe. In post-colonial Zimbabwe, the government introduced several changes to hospital spaces. These included dismantling colonial policies and in the process opening up hospitals to Zimbabweans of all races and social classes. The government also accelerated the Africanisation of key structures within the hospital system and nursing services. In addition, the government improved nurses' working conditions. However, hospitals continued to experience numerous challenges inherited from the colonial period, namely, lack of investment and, for the nurses, increased workloads.

The situation took a massive turn in the early 1990s when the government adopted austerity measures. The introduction of ESAP resulted in a reduction in government investment in the public sector, which also led to a decline in the budget allocation for public hospitals and negatively affected the nurses' capacity to provide services to patients. At the same time, the emergence of the HIV/AIDS menace, at a time when nurses were working with limited resources, complicated the situation. Working conditions deteriorated, real wages declined and nurses experienced increased workloads by the mid-1990s.

Nurses were not passive victims of their situation. They employed various strategies to cope with the changing working environment. Some nurses joined the private sector or migrated abroad, while the majority remained in the public sector – providing medical care. Some of the forms of agency exhibited by public hospital nurses included buying their own protective gear, using second/third rate drugs in the face of drug shortages and restricting admissions in an attempt to reduce a surge in patient numbers. Furthermore, some nurses started various business activities such as cross-border trading in order to supplement their salaries.

The most controversial of all responses was the industrial action evidenced by the 1996 public sector strikes, led by nurses. An examination of the strikes exposed the tensions within the nursing fraternity. The strikes seemed to deviate from the traditional notions of nursing as a vocation vis-à-vis a profession. While authorities emphasised the nature of the profession and patients' rights in their response to the strikes, the nurses argued that the industrial action route was not a betrayal of the oath to save lives. Rather, the nurses positioned themselves as workers who were requesting the government to improve the health-care system and, as activists, demanding the right to determine the most conducive way to effectively execute their duty to the community.

Notes

1 The first decade of independence witnessed Zimbabwe making tremendous progress in the provision of health facilities and quality services to the majority of its citizens. Infant and maternal health statistics are good indicators of this progress. For instance, 83% of Zimbabwean children were immunised against measles and other childhood diseases by 1990. This Zimbabwean success was second only to Mauritius in Africa. Furthermore, the country had the lowest rate of childhood malnutrition in Sub-Saharan Africa, and the child mortality rate was less than half the African average of 88 per 1,000, and maternal mortality rate was only 251 per 100,000 births. The World Bank acknowledged and praised these remarkable strides in quality health care provision. For more, see Mlambo, *The Economic Structural Adjustment Programme*, p. 2.
2 See Marks, *Divided sisterhood*.
3 H. M. S. Ushewokunze, 'Primary health care for Zimbabwe. What does it mean?': Lunchtime meeting of National Affairs Association, Anglican Cathedral Hall, Friday 20 March 1981, in H. S. M. Ushwewokunze, *An agenda for Zimbabwe* (Harare: College Press, 1984), pp. 109–21.
4 S. T. Agere, 'Progress and problems in the health care', in I. Mandaza (ed.), *Zimbabwe: The political economy of transition, 1980–1986* (Dakar: Codesria, 1986), pp. 355–76.
5 Ushewokunze, 'Primary Health Care for Zimbabwe', pp. 109–21.
6 J. Gillmurray, R. Riddel and D. Sanders, *The struggles for health from Rhodesia to Zimbabwe* (London: Catholic Institute for International Relations, 1979), p. 37.
7 For more on Equity in Health see R. Loewenson, D. Sanders and R. Davies, 'Challenges to equity in health and health care: A Zimbabwean case study', *Social Science & Medicine*, 32: 10 (1991), pp. 1079–88.

8 'Health', in ZANU-PF, *Zimbabwe at 5 years of independence: Achievements, problems and prospects* (Preface: R. G. Mugabe) (Harare: ZANU (PF) Department of Commissariat and Culture, 1985), pp. 189–224.
9 NAZ MS 308/38/6. Health During the Liberation Struggle, British Broadcasting Corporation (Text report), 16 September 1980.
10 NAZ MS 308/38/6. Health During the Liberation Struggle, British Broadcasting Corporation (Text report), 16 September 1980.
11 NAZ MS 308/38/6. Health During the Liberation Struggle, Ministry of Health Statement on Zimbabwe's Proposed Free Health Services, 30 August 1980.
12 D. Sanders, 'Equity in Health: Zimbabwe Nine Years On', *Journal of Social Development in Africa*, 5: 1 (1990) 5–22.
13 Sanders, 'Equity in health: Zimbabwe nine years on'.
14 The Hospital Services Act was an act that legislated 'open' (white only) and 'closed' (black only) hospitals. The repeal of the act meant that former white only hospitals like Andrew Fleming Hospital and United Bulawayo Hospitals for example, removed restrictions on African patients.
15 Interview: Mrs E. Mawoyo, Chikanga Mutare, 22 February 2009.
16 *The Herald*, 25 October 1980.
17 *The Herald*, 25 October 1980.
18 Ushewokunze, *An agenda for Zimbabwe*, p. 125.
19 Jackson, *Surfacing up*, p. 185.
20 Interview Mrs Nomsa Makoni, Chitungwiza, 20 April 2009.
21 Jackson, *Surfacing up*, p. 185.
22 Jackson, *Surfacing up*, p. 185.
23 Interview: Mrs Nomsa Makoni, Chitungwiza, 20 April 2009.
24 NAZ MS 308/38/6. Health During the Liberation Struggle.
25 ZANLA (Zimbabwe National Liberation Army) was the armed wing of the ruling party ZANU (PF) party.
26 G. Chidyausiku (ZANU PF) *Zimbabwe Parliamentary Debates*, Vol. 2, 1980–1981, 19 August to 8 October 1980, 20 January to 7 May 1981.
27 G. Chidyausiku (ZANU PF) *Zimbabwe Parliamentary Debates*, Vol. 2, 1980–1981, 19 August to 8 October 1980, 20 January to 7 May 1981.
28 From 23–25 November 1977, the Rhodesian Security Forces bombed two refugee camps in Mozambique at Chimoio and Tembwe. More than 3,000 refugees and members of ZANLA, the armed wing of ZANU (PF), were killed.
29 *The Sunday Mail*, 14 September 1980.
30 *The Sunday Mail*, 14 September 1980.
31 The Republican Front (renamed 1981) was the successor of the Rhodesian Front led by Ian Smith. In the 1980 election, the RF won all twenty parliamentary seats reserved for whites. In 1984 the RF became the Conservative Alliance of Zimbabwe. Eleven of its twenty parliamentarians defected over the following four years, but the party again won fifteen of the twenty

parliamentary seats reserved for whites in the 1985 election. In 1987 the ruling government abolished all reserved seats for whites. When these were abolished many white MPs became independents or joined the ruling ZANU (PF) party.
32 R. Cronje (Republican Front) *Zimbabwe Parliamentary Debates*, Vol. 2, 1980-1981, 19 August to 8 October 1980, 20 January to 7 May 1981.
33 W. D. Walker (Republican Front) *Zimbabwe Parliamentary Debates*, Vol. 2, 1980-1981, 19 August to 8 October 1980, 20 January to 7 May 1981.
34 R. Cartwright (Republican Front) *Zimbabwe Parliamentary Debates*, Vol. 2, 1980-1981, 19 August to 8 October 1980, 20 January to 7 May 1981.
35 G. Chidyausiku (ZANU PF) *Zimbabwe Parliamentary Debates*, Vol. 2, 1980-1981, 19 August to 8 October 1980, 20 January to 7 May 1981.
36 Chidyausiku (ZANU PF) *Zimbabwe Parliamentary Debates*.
37 Chidyausiku (ZANU PF) *Zimbabwe Parliamentary Debates*.
38 H. Ushewokunze (ZANU PF) *Zimbabwe Parliamentary Debates*, Vol. 2, 1980-1981, 19 August to 8 October 1980, 20 January to 7 May 1981.
39 Interview: Mrs Doreen Mabika, Palmerstone Mutare, 4 January 2009.
40 ZANU-PF, 'Health', *Zimbabwe at 5 years of independence*, pp. 189-224.
41 ZANU-PF, 'Health', *Zimbabwe at 5 years of independence*, pp. 189-224
42 Interview: Mrs Nomsa Makoni, Chitungwiza, 20 April 2009.
43 Interview: Mrs Nomsa Makoni, Chitungwiza, 20 April 2009.
44 Interview: Mrs Nelia Ncube, Chitungwiza, 20 April 2009.
45 Interview: Mrs Nelia Ncube, Chitungwiza, 20 April 2009.
46 Interview: Mrs Maida Tsopora, Harare, 28 October 2008.
47 *The Sunday Mail*, 11 December 1983.
48 Mrs Marere quoted in I. Mhike, 'A perennial shortage: State Registered Nurse training and recruitment in Southern Rhodesia's government hospitals, 1939-1963' (MA dissertation, University of Zimbabwe, 2007), p. 89.
49 Mrs Hadebe quoted in C. Govha, 'A Study of the implications of racial and gender prejudices on African women in the Nursing Profession in Colonial Zimbabwe, 1890-1960' (BA Honours dissertation, University of Zimbabwe, 2001), p. 29.
50 N. Khan and N. Jazdowska, 'Women, workers and discrimination in Zimbabwe', in B. Raftopoulos and L. Sachikonye (eds), *Striking back: The labour movement and the post-colonial state in Zimbabwe, 1980-2000* (Harare, Weaver Press, 2001) pp. 175-96.
51 P. A. Made and N. Whande, 'Women in Southern Africa: A note on the Zimbabwean "success story"', *Issue: A Journal of Opinion*, 17: 2 (1989), pp. 26-8.
52 Interview: Mrs Makoni, Chitungwiza, 20 April 2009.
53 *Moto*, June 1981.
54 *The Sunday Mail*, 11 December 1983.
55 Interview: Mrs Makoni, Chitungwiza, 20 April 2009.

56 A. S. Mlambo, *The Economic Structural Adjustment Programme: The case of Zimbabwe, 1990–1995* (Harare: UZ Publications, 1997), p. 79.
57 Mlambo, *The Economic Structural Adjustment Programme*, p. 79.
58 Mlambo, *The Economic Structural Adjustment Programme*, p. 79.
59 Mlambo, *The Economic Structural Adjustment Programme*, p. 2.
60 Mlambo, *The Economic Structural Adjustment Programme*, p. 2.
61 L. A. Bijlmakers, M. T. Bassett and D. M. Sanders, 'Health and Structural Adjustment in rural and urban settings in Zimbabwe: Some interim findings', in P. Gibbon (ed.), *Structural Adjustment and the working poor* (Uppsala: Nordiska Africainstitutet, 1995), pp. 215–82.
62 Bijlmakers, Bassett and Sanders, 'Health and Structural Adjustment', pp. 215–82.
63 Mlambo, *The Economic Structural Adjustment Programme*, p. 86.
64 Interviews with Mrs Laiza Shumba, Mabelreign, Harare, 26 October 2008; Mrs Dumbura, Mufakose, Harare, 22 October 2008; Ms Tsitsi Chinamasa, Old Mutare, 28 May 2009; Mrs Nomsa Makoni, Chitungwiza, 20 April 2009; Mrs Nelia Ncube, Chitungwiza, 20 April 2009.
65 Mlambo, *The Economic Structural Adjustment Programme*, p. 86.
66 Interviews: Mrs Viola Moyo, Harare, 20 November 2008; Mrs Laiza Shumba, Mabelreign, Harare, 26 October 2008.
67 Interview: Ms Claris Bere, Harare, July 2009. Interview by P. Mukwambo.
68 D. Mutizwa-Mangiza, *Doctors and the state: The struggle for professional control* (Aldershot: Ashgate, 1999), p. 117.
69 Interview: Ms Claris Bere, Harare, July 2009. Interview by P. Mukwambo.
70 The Zimbabwe Nurses Association (ZINA) is a voluntary organisation that represents nurses. It formed in 1981 to replace the Southern Rhodesia Nurses Association, an organisation that primarily represented the interests of white nurses during the colonial period.
71 Sr Clara Nondo, quoted in *The Worker*, February 1994.
72 Interview: Mrs Flora Matondo, Sakubva Mutare, August 2008.
73 *The Worker*, March 1996. Interviews also corroborated this report and explained that shortages of food at hospitals was something they have never experienced since they started working.
74 *The Worker*, March 1996.
75 Report of the Secretary for Health and Child Welfare for the year ending 31 December 1994, p. 15.
76 S. Ray and F. Madzimbamuto. 'The HIV Epidemic in Zimbabwe: The penalty of silence', *The Round Table*, 95: 384 (2006), pp. 219–38.
77 Ray and Madzimbamuto. 'The HIV epidemic in Zimbabwe', pp. 219–38.
78 Interview: Mrs Doreen Mabika, Palmerstone Mutare, 4 January 2009.
79 For contemporary problems with HIV exposure, see for example, J. Zelnick and M. O'Donnell, 'The impact of HIV/AIDS Epidemic on hospital nurses

in KwaZulu Natal, South Africa', *Journal of Public Health Policy*, 26 (2005), pp. 163–85.
80 *The Worker*, February 1994.
81 Dr P. L. N. Sikosana, Secretary for Health and Child Welfare to Dr T. Stamps, Minister of Health and Child Welfare, Report of the Secretary for Health and Child Welfare for the year ending 31 December 1995, p. 2.
82 Interview: Mrs Jane Mushando, Sakubva Mutare, 27 April 2009.
83 Dr P. L. N. Sikosana, Secretary for Health and Child Welfare to Dr T. Stamps, Minister of Health and Child Welfare, Report of the Secretary for Health and Child Welfare for the year ending 31 December 1996.
84 D. P. L. N. Sikosana, Secretary for Health and Child Welfare to Dr T. Stamps, Minister of Health and Child Welfare, Report of the Secretary for Health and Child Welfare for the year ending 31 December 1998.
85 The Director of Nursing claimed that the public health sector was losing about 10 per cent of the total every year. Most of the nurses migrated to Botswana, South Africa, the UK and Australia. For more see, Gaidzanwa, *Voting with their feet*.
86 Interview Mrs Nomsa Makoni, Chitungwiza, 20 April 2009.
87 Bijlmakers, Bassett and Sanders, 'Health and Structural Adjustment', pp. 215–82.
88 Bijlmakers, Bassett and Sanders, 'Health and Structural Adjustment', pp. 215–82.
89 Interview: Mbuya Veronica Sibanda, Harare, 15 September 2008.
90 *National Observer*, 28 December 1978.
91 Interview: Ms Claris Bere, Harare, July 2009. Interview by P. Mukwambo.
92 Interview: Mrs Jane Mushando, Sakubva Mutare, 27 April 2009.
93 A patient quoted in Bijlmakers, Bassett and Sanders, 'Health and Structural Adjustment', pp. 215–82.
94 Mlambo, *The Economic Structural Adjustment Programme*, p. 84.
95 For a discussion on nurses and their struggle to enter the so-called middle class, see Chapter 3 and for other countries such as South Africa see Horwitz, *Baragwanath Hospital*.
96 The private hospital sector became the preferred destination for most nurses as it offered a number of advantages. Not only were salaries pegged according to inflation and adjusted regularly, it also meant less stress and disruption to family on the part of the nurses. However, the private sector would only accommodate a small percentage of highly skilled and experienced nurses. Thus, others decided to vote with their feet and went in search of greener pastures within the region and abroad.
97 Historically, African associations were established in urban areas during the colonial period in response to the economic conditions faced by Africans during the era. Women would come together to organise feasts, funerals and other informal associations, and these activities constituted the survival strategies that informed urban women's strategies. See, for example, A. M. Tripp, 'Deindustrialization and the growth of women's economic associations and

networks in urban Tanzania', in S. Rowbotham and S. Mitter (eds), *Dignity and daily bread: New forms of economic organising among poor women in the third world and the first* (London: Penguin, 1994), pp. 139–57.
98 See for example, Ennie Chipembere, 'Cross-border trade: A coping mechanism adopted by Zimbabweans: A case study of Harare 1980–1999' (BA Honours Dissertation, University of Zimbabwe, 1999).
99 Interview: Mrs Etella Dhlamini, Harare, 22 August 2008.
100 Interview: Mrs Etella Dhlamini, Harare, 22 August 2008.
101 Bijlmakers, Bassett and Sanders, 'Health and Structural Adjustment', pp. 215–82.
102 For South Africa see N. Lubanga, 'Nursing in South Africa: Black women workers organize', in M. Turshen (ed.), *Women and health in Africa* (Trenton: Africa World Press, 1991), pp. 51–77.
103 Melosh, *The physician's hand*, p. 199.
104 Interview: Mrs Estella Dhlamini, Harare, 22 August 2008.
105 Marks, *Divided sisterhood*.
106 Interview: Mrs Viola Moyo, Harare, 20 November 2008.
107 *The Herald*, 22 October 1996.
108 *The Herald*, 22 October 1996.
109 *The Herald*, 22 October 1996.
110 *The Herald*, 22 October 1996.
111 Interview: Mbuya Veronica Sibanda, Harare, 15 September 2008.
112 *The Herald*, 23 October 1996.
113 Interview: Mbuya Veronica Sibanda, Harare, 15 September 2008.
114 Interview: Mbuya Veronica Sibanda, Harare, 15 September 2008.
115 *The Herald*, 31 October 1996.
116 *The Herald*, 31 October 1996.
117 Interview: Mbuya Veronica Sibanda, Harare, 15 September 2008.
118 *The Herald*, 21 November 1996.
119 *The Herald*, 15 November 1996.
120 See Melosh, *The physician's hand*.
121 *The Herald*, 31 October 1996.
122 *The Herald*, 1 November 1996.
123 *The Herald*, 31 October 1996.
124 *The Herald*, 31 October 1996.
125 *The Herald*, 30 October 1996.
126 *The Herald*, 31 October 1996. LOMA stands for Law and Order Maintenance Act, a draconian law that was passed in 1960 and was a legislative tool aimed at stifling dissent against white minority rule. The bill remained intact until it was replaced by another draconian bill called the Public Order and Security Act (POSA) in 2002.
127 *The Zimbabwe Independent*, 15–21 November 1996.

128 Mrs M. Chidzonga, Member of Parliament, *Zimbabwe Parliamentary Debates*, 27 November 1996.
129 Ms M. Dongo, Member of Parliament, *Zimbabwe Parliamentary Debates*, 27 November 1996.
130 Mr R. Shambambeva-Nyandoro, Member of Parliament, *Zimbabwe Parliamentary Debates*, 27 November 1996.
131 *The Herald*, 23 October 1996.
132 R. Sanders, 'Striking ahead: Industrial action and labour movement development in Zimbabwe', in B. Raftopoulos and L. Sachikonye (eds), *Striking back: The labour movement and post-colonial state in Zimbabwe* (Harare: Weaver Press, 2001), pp. 133–74.
133 *The Herald*, 12 November 1996.
134 *The Sunday Mail*, 10 November 1996.
135 Interview: Mrs Nomsa Makoni, Chitungwiza, 20 April 2009.
136 *The Herald*, 31 October 1996.
137 *The Sunday Mail*, 10 November 1996.
138 Interviews: Mrs Nomsa Makoni, Chitungwiza, 20 April 2009. Mrs Estella Dhlamini, Harare, 22 August 2008.
139 *The Sunday Mail*, 17 November 1996.
140 Interviews: Mrs Nomsa Makoni, Chitungwiza, 20 April 2009 and Mrs Estella Dhlamini, Harare, 22 August 2008.
141 Dr P. L. N. Sikosana, Secretary for Health and Child Welfare to Dr T. Stamps, Minister of Health and Child Welfare, Report of the Secretary for Health and Child Welfare, for the year ending 31 December 1996.

7
Conclusion: Nurses and nursing in twentieth-century Zimbabwe

The image (Figure 7.1) shows an African leprosy patient and two nurses – an African and a European in the dispensary. The African nurse, in a dark dress and wearing gloves, is treating the leprosy patient. The white nurse, in a white uniform, is most likely instructing the African nurse on where to apply medicine. The image is about a teaching moment as much as it demonstrates a healing process. It also reveals the relations between the patient and the healers, and the healers themselves – black and white. It is about a colonial institution – the clinic – that was to transform the healing landscape in twentieth-century Zimbabwe. Plucked in time, the image also sums up the nature of work and the people who dispensed medicine within Zimbabwe's hospitals for close to a century. The African nurse, with the guidance of the European nurse – even with the Africanisation that began in the 1960s onwards – remained the central figure in dispensing biomedicine to her fellow African patients. It is, therefore, a story that undergirds this book – the African nurse and everyday work in Zimbabwe's hospitals in the twentieth century.

I examine the role of African health-care workers in their different capacities within government hospitals in colonial and post-colonial Zimbabwe. In the process, I delineate the history of the hospital system in Zimbabwe over the twentieth century. Starting with the early medical auxiliaries recruited by missionaries during the first decade of the twentieth century, I demonstrate the importance of these men and women to the functioning of the makeshift hospitals. Sometimes classified as nursing orderlies and sometimes referred to as medical orderlies, these men and women embraced the opportunities

Conclusion

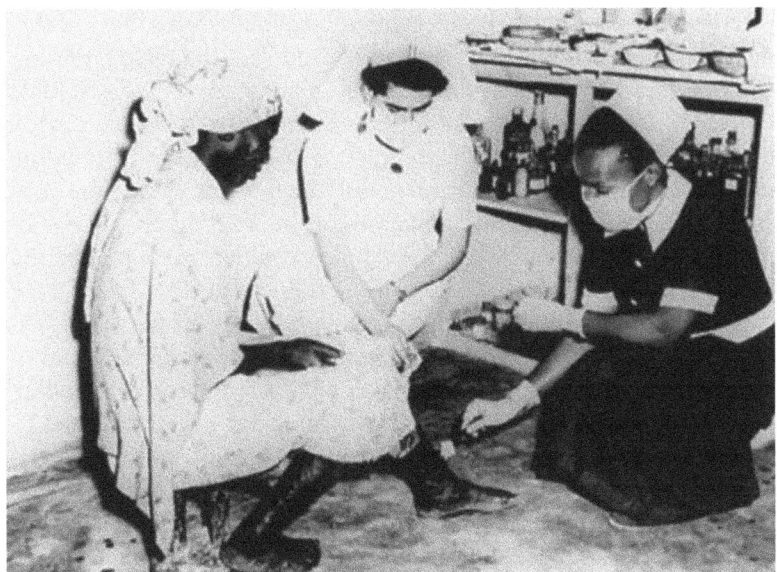

Figure 7.1 Treatment of leprosy (courtesy National Archives of Zimbabwe)

presented to them by the missionaries, mining companies and later on by the government, not only to improve their lives, but also to dispense medical services to their fellow Africans. The early generation of medical auxiliaries, just like the later generation of nurses, fought disease and nursed the infirm. By highlighting the roles of early medical auxiliaries, I do not propose that they were tools of colonial medicine, and neither do I present a celebratory account of these hospital workers. On the contrary, by historicising early medical orderlies' experiences, I suggest a need for scholars to appreciate the various ways early nursing orderlies provided services in demanding conditions. They worked with limited resources in rudimentary hospitals. They inherited the disease world of the late nineteenth century. They tackled new medical conditions as the capitalist economy expanded, just as they encountered new diseases like influenza.

Mission nurses followed the paths trodden by the early medical auxiliaries. Started at Waddilove Mission by Sr Dry, by the mid-1940s numerous mission stations scattered across Rhodesia were training young women as nurses. Besides mission-trained nurses, the government also began training its version of a nurse – the male orderlies. The orderlies staffed rural clinics and hospitals across Rhodesia. Male orderlies, together with mission nurses, carried on the work started by the early medical auxiliaries, nursing the infirm and providing medical care to Africans in rural areas. The mission nurses and government orderlies laid the foundation for the training of a variety of medical auxiliaries including government-trained midwives in the 1940s. A significant shift came with the training of the African State Registered Nurses, also known as qualified nurses, in the 1950s. Up until the time the government began considering the possibilities of training African SRNs, the category of SRN was a preserve for white women.[1] For various reasons, though, Rhodesia never managed to train enough white SRNs. By the late 1930s and into the 1940s, the colony was experiencing a shortage of white SRNs.[2] The urbanisation of Africans from the 1930s onwards stretched service delivery in urban hospitals. Hence, Europeans and non-Europeans alike called on the government to train African, coloured and Asian SRNs to cater to their communities. For various reasons, SRN training focused on women and excluded men. It was not until 1966 that the government commenced the training of male SRNs.[3] For the largest part of the second half of the twentieth century, save for the 1970s with the introduction of the guerrilla medic at the height of the liberation war, the female African SRN remained pivotal to the hospital system.

The centrality of the African to the hospital system is undeniable. By the beginning of the second decade of the twentieth century, medical auxiliaries such as Job Tsiga, Jonathan Manyoka and David Sakutomba together with a host of nursing maids had demonstrated their importance in the provision of nursing and medical services to many Africans who sought medical treatment at mission stations. The early medical auxiliaries transformed western healing spaces into their own. Government-trained nursing orderlies, as well as nurses who took up the profession from the post-Second World War period, continued this transformation to the extent that by the 1950s onwards, Africans constituted the majority of hospital workers. Even when they were the majority, for the entire period of colonial rule, African nurses were subordinates to their white counterparts.

Conclusion

Through privileging the experiences of the subordinates, I use the case of healing spaces to examine colonial relations. I argue that hospital relations replicated larger social relations. As in South Africa, the structure and organisation of hospital bureaucracy reflected the broader societal structures.[4] At the top of the pyramid were hospital administrators and medical doctors, followed by white nurses. At the base of the pyramid were African nurses who bore the weight of tending the infirm. Even in the post-colonial period, with the completion of the Africanisation of the hospital system, the structure of the hospital remained very much a colonial one. Black hospital administrators, black matrons and sisters in charge perpetuated the former hospital relations, as was done in the past – with the majority of nurses constituting the fulcrum of the smooth functioning of the hospital system. In shouldering the burden of hospital work over the twentieth century, African nurses in their various categories and generations, female or male, used the opportunity to carve a niche for themselves within Zimbabwean hospitals. In the process, they made clinical spaces their own. African nurses used their presence in hospitals to highlight their potential and expertise. Early medical auxiliaries, nursing orderlies, SRNs and guerrilla medics were bastions of the healing spaces they controlled. And beyond the gaze and reach of officials and superiors – whether as Advanced Male Native Nursing Orderlies of the 1930s and 1940s, junior nurses from the 1950s onwards, Advanced Clinical Nurses in the 1970s, or as guerrilla medics – these various types of nurses became de facto medical authorities. This is significant for nursing history. As de facto medical authorities, nurses had control over their work and yielded power within the clinic and beyond the clinic: the power that was elusive to many an African during the long twentieth century. They acquired knowledge associated with biomedicine, diagnosed disease and made decisions on the nature of treatment. Even if it meant referring patients to the next nursing or medical authority higher on the chain of command, it was in itself a demonstration of authority on nursing and medical issues that was a privilege of the few. In addition, as de facto authorities within clinical spaces, nurses in their various capacities also blurred the boundaries between nursing practice and medical work.

I highlight the significance of African nurses' intermediary position within healing spaces. While African nurses were not tools of biomedical practices, they nonetheless made it easy for African patients to adjust to clinical experiences. As cultural interlocutors, African nurses were central in translating African conceptions of afflictions to white medical personnel, simultaneously translating western medicine to African patients. It was nurses' responsibility to acquire the correct information for doctors and to make the diagnosis easier.[5] African nurses' presence within hospitals reassured many patients that they were being served by their own people. Toward this end, nurses drew upon their cultural understanding of disease causation in helping patients comprehend and negotiate different healthcare options.[6] As in other parts of the continent, African nurses during the twentieth century played a pivotal role as cultural brokers between Africans and Europeans within clinical spaces.[7] As cultural interlocutors, African nurses were central in shaping how the afflicted experienced colonial medicine, even though they enjoyed less authority and power than their European counterparts.

Closely related to the above, I stress the idea that the sphere of nursing became an arena in which Africans reshaped western and African meanings of care-giving, and at the same time reformulated the local care economy.[8] The hospital environment enabled nurses to cross the cultural nursing boundaries, in the process reshaping Africans' understanding of taking care of the sick and tending the infirm. For example, through an examination of young women's experiences in the post-1950 period, I demonstrate how young African nurses adjusted to seeing strangers' bodies, especially male bodies, as well as probing healthy and diseased body parts as part of their work. Furthermore, I note how nursing older patients presented a major cultural challenge to young African women. With time, nurses got used to the changes. Thus, while young nurses pushed the boundaries of traditional understandings of nursing through their presence in clinical spaces, the normalisation of their earlier anxieties was one of the ways in which African nurses reshaped their cultural understandings of nursing.

It is important to note that the segregationist and racist policies that were the hallmark of Rhodesian society extended to clinical spaces.[9] Besides racially segregating hospitals, Rhodesian authorities

Conclusion

prohibited African nurses from tending white patients in government hospitals.[10] While this policy worked for most of the colonial period, the policy came under scrutiny in the twilight of the colonial era. Faced with shortages of white nurses in the 1970s, some sections of the white community were bent on preserving racial privileges and racial segregation within clinical spaces, just as they were fighting nationalists to maintain the hallmarks of Rhodesian society. The closure of white wards at Bindura Hospital due to the shortages of white nurses and the continued defence of the policy that restricted Africans from nursing white patients, were reminders of the authorities' determination to limit racial contact in hospitals.[11] Racial segregation within clinical spaces in the 1970s exposed anxieties amongst Rhodesians.[12]

Skirted in nursing history is an examination of nurses' hopes and aspirations for choosing the profession. I fill this gap in the historiography. As noted, earlier generations of nurses took advantage of the opportunities presented by the presence of new healing spaces to improve themselves, and so did the later generations of nurses. The fact that the government opened nursing to African women due to structural changes in Rhodesia in the 1940s did not mean that African women were not able to imagine the possibilities offered by the nursing profession. I highlight that in an environment that limited women's opportunities because of their gender and race, African women used nursing as a ladder to secure a better life for themselves and their families. For those who entered the nursing programme, their new careers transformed their lives and contributed to the sudden and unprecedented rise in their social positions in an oppressive society. Nursing gave them a sense of their competency and allowed them to contribute to society in ways that would have been impossible for many. Public spaces like hospitals and clinics became new sites that African women used to reshape and negotiate social relations and move up the social ladder. Christine Mawema captured the potential offered by the professionalisation of women in Rhodesia when she said: 'Our kitchen days are over … We can no longer continue the tradition of our predecessors. We just want to be treated as equals with our men and we will do it, I tell you!'[13] The wife of Nelson Mawema, one of the early nationalists in African politics, Christine Mawema, saw Africans' struggle to be treated with dignity as part of women's struggle.[14] Therefore, I use the professionalisation of African women as a window into examining how African women's everyday lives were no longer being defined by their domestic responsibilities and by their association to men, either as suitors, husbands or their male relatives, but by their newfound status as professional women. In the process, I bridge the divide between the private and public spheres – an understudied theme in nursing history.

Lastly, I extend the parameters of nursing history by examining the experiences of nurses in the first sixteen years of independence. I explore the steps taken by the government to improve nurses' working conditions. The government completed the Africanisation of the hospital hierarchy. While there were notable changes to nurses' working conditions, the old problems experienced in the colonial period endured. Huge workloads and the unavailability of resources continued to frustrate nurses. Even with the persistence of the problems inherited from the colonial period, one can observe what looks like a pretty straightforward esprit-de-corps among nurses for the most part of the first decade of independence. This must be understood within the euphoria surrounding the 1980s due to Zimbabwe's independence. In the 1980s, nurses, just as the rest of the society, felt it was their duty to nurse the new nation. Hence the past struggles were used as motivating factors to provide services to their fellow Africans. But this euphoria was a fleeting one. The esprit-de-corps among nurses faded by the end of the 1980s decade as nurses, just as their predecessors, began to strongly criticise the government's failure to improve their working conditions.

In fact, the situation took a major turn in the early 1990s when the government implemented the Economic Structural Adjustment Programme, thus reducing investment in the public health sector. At the same time, the emergence of HIV/AIDS worsened the state of affairs within hospitals. In their subordinate position, just like their predecessors, nurses adapted to the situation creatively. To supplement their salaries, some nurses became involved in various business activities such as cross-border trading. In response to declining working conditions, nurses resorted to work slowdowns, confrontations with administrators and at times, open protests and strikes.

I demonstrate that as a counter to nurses' coping strategies, hospital administrators and the government emphasised the nature of

Conclusion

the profession. Nurses argued that they had to continue tending to the sick irrespective of the challenges at hand. Officials also rallied behind patients' rights. I note that the various strategies deployed by nurses did not mean a negation of their responsibilities to patients and society, as state officials and hospital administrators argued. Instead, by adopting the tactics mentioned earlier, nurses showed a profound responsibility to patients, commitment to their work and the desire to provide the best care to Zimbabweans. As important historical actors, nurses went beyond expectations in their efforts to seek to redress the declining working standards. As workers demanded that the government improve the health-care system, nurses demanded the right to determine the best way to satisfy their duty to the community.

The history of nurses has been neglected within Zimbabwean historiography. I try to fill part of this gap. While examining the experiences of African nurses in great detail, this is not a definitive history of nurses in Zimbabwe. There is still more to be written about the countless men and women who, for over a century, stood on the frontline of providing medical care to millions of Zimbabweans. I hope that my work will stimulate other under-researched issues within nursing history in Zimbabwe as well as within the Southern African region and beyond. The inclusion of such Southern African perspectives will broaden the scope of global nursing history.

There are three major themes that require further research in Zimbabwe's nursing history. These are gender, race and the role of professional nursing organisations. In Zimbabwe, as in the rest of Southern Africa, nursing historiography has mainly paid attention to female nurses. The focus on female nurses is not surprising, considering that the majority of nurses are women. However, there have been several male nurses since the inception of the hospital system. Some research has already been conducted on this topic in Southern Africa. South African historians, Burns and Marks examine the presence of male nurses in South Africa within the context of mining and the war.[15] Besides writing men into nursing history, Burns and Marks' works explore discourses around masculinity and appropriate careers.[16] In this book, I demonstrate the presence of male medical orderlies who practised nursing in government and mission hospitals and highlight the role of guerrilla medics who were central in the provision of medical services to freedom fighters during the 1970s war.[17] Still, in Zimbabwe, the male SRNs was a rare species until the middle of the 1960s, when the government commenced the training of male SRNs. For those interested in male nurses, it will be essential to examine the reasons for this change in policy on the part of the government, why these men took up the profession, which, for the most part, was dominated by women, as well as to understand how male nurses interacted with their female colleagues. In examining the history of male nursing, I urge scholars to move beyond mining and the war – which have traditionally been dominated by men and thus can be considered as male spaces – by exploring the experiences of male nurses in ordinary hospitals. An analysis of male nursing outside the ambit of mining and the military in Zimbabwe and Southern Africa will further complicate the discourse around nursing and masculinities within nursing historiography.

In this book, I pay attention to African nurses. Yet during the twentieth century, professional nurses had diverse racial backgrounds. In Zimbabwe, the first hospital nurses were white Dominican Sisters under the guidance of Mother Patrick. The sisters were replaced by white lay nurses at the turn of the twentieth century.[18] White nurses remained a constant factor in the history of nurses, yet there is less discussion of them in the literature.[19] Furthermore, I hardly examine coloured nurses and nurses of Asian descent. A more comprehensive history of nurses in Zimbabwe and in extension, Southern Africa should include these racial clusters as the history of African nurses is incomplete without further examining their interactions with these groups. The inclusion of other races in nursing history can be used as a point of entry into examining similarities and differences in experiences for nurses based on race across time and space.

An area that I skirt round in this book is professional nurses' organisations. Nurses, just like other workers, organised to fight for their rights and influence policies that affected their daily work within hospitals.[20] Hence an examination of the networks created by organisations representing nurses and labour movements is another area that needs to be further researched. Indeed, nursing is mostly perceived as an elite profession that has less in common with the rest of the workforce. Yet, as the analysis of the 1996 strikes has demonstrated, the nursing profession is not immune to the problems

Conclusion

affecting the rest of the workforce. A study of nurses and the broader workforce unsettle the narrative that projects nurses as elites, blurring and complicating the seeming boundaries between nurses and other workers. An investigation of these and possible other neglected issues in nursing history will add a further layer to the role of nurses in the history of Zimbabwe, the region and the world.

Informed by the memories of nurses, I highlight the experiences of men and women, trained and untrained nurses, mission nurses and government nurses, orderlies and guerrilla medics. In their various capacities and within the different healing spaces in which they worked, these healthcare workers transformed the hospitals to make them their own. In the process, they reshaped and reformulated indigenous as well as western nursing and biomedical practices. Through their work, they contributed to the development of the nation by being at the bedside, healing the sick and nursing the infirm.

Notes

1 Masakure, 'One of the most serious problems'.
2 Masakure, 'One of the most serious problems'.
3 Report of the Secretary for Health for the year ending 31 December 1966.
4 Marks, *Divided sisterhood*; Horwitz, *Baragwanath Hospital*; Burns, 'A man is too clumsy a thing who does not know how to handle a sick person', pp. 695–717.
5 Interview: Mrs Matondo, Sakubva Mutare, 12 August 2009; Mrs Nyaradzo Buzengwe, Harare, 10 July 2009; Mrs Shumba, Mabelreign Harare, 26 October 2008.
6 Interview: Mrs Matondo, Sakubva Mutare, 12 August 2009; Mrs Nyaradzo Buzengwe, Harare, 10 July 2009; Mrs Shumba, Mabelreign Harare, 26 October 2008.
7 For other parts of Africa see for example, Digby and Sweet, 'Nurses as cultural brokers in twentieth-century South Africa', pp. 113–29; Hunt, *A colonial lexicon*; Vaughan, *Curing their ills*; Kalusa, 'Language, medical auxiliaries', pp. 57–78; Turritin, 'Colonial midwives and modernizing childbirth in French West Africa', pp. 71–91.
8 For East Africa, see for example, Illife, *East African doctors* and White, *Speaking with vampires*.
9 Levy, 'Keeping abreast of the times', pp. 158–9.
10 NAZ MS 308/38/2 Health Services in Relation to the Liberation Struggle, newspaper cutting from. *The Rhodesia Herald*, 21 November 1974.
11 *The Rhodesia Herald*, 22 January 1975.

12 *The Rhodesia Herald*, 22 January 1975; *The Rhodesia Herald*, 25 January 1975; R. T. D. Sadomba, *Rhodesia Parliamentary Debates*, vol. 91, 5–29 August 1975; Dr Barlow (MP, Avondale) *Rhodesia Parliamentary Debates*, vol. 91, 5–29 August 1975.
13 *The African Parade*, December 1960.
14 *The African Parade*, December 1960.
15 See Marks, 'We were men nursing men', pp. 177–204 and Burns, 'A man is a clumsy thing who does not know how to handle a sick person', pp. 695–717.
16 See Marks, 'We were men nursing men', pp. 177–204 and Burns, 'A man is a clumsy thing who does not know how to handle a sick person', pp. 695–717.
17 See Chapter 2 and Chapter 5.
18 See Charumbira, 'Administering medicine without a license' and Gelfand, *Tropical victory*.
19 See Masakure, 'One of the most serious problems' and Mhike, 'A perennial shortage'.
20 For Zimbabwe, I am thinking of organisations such as the South African Trained Nurses Association, the Rhodesia Nurses Association and its successor the Zimbabwe Nurses Association.

Appendix 1

Colonial and post-colonial names

Colonial names	Post-colonial names
Andrew Fleming Hospital	Parirenyatwa Hospital
Gwelo	Gweru
Harari Hospital	Harare Hospital
Harari Township	Mbare Township
Impilo Hospital	Mpilo Hospital
Old Umtali	Old Mutare
Rhodesia	Zimbabwe
Salisbury	Harare
Umtali	Mutare
Mtoko	Mutoko
Mrewa	Murehwa

Appendix 2

Explanations and translations

chipotswa	An affliction characterized by the sensation of an object moving rhythmically from one part of the body to another, for example from the left ear to the right groin. It is believed that that the affliction is a result of bewitchment.
chirungu/chingezi	Westernisation.
coloured	I use the term coloured to refer to people of mixed race. This is a popular term that is used throughout Southern Africa.
kufunda	Education.
kuroyiwa	Witchcraft.
lurwara	Getting sick.
Location	In colonial Zimbabwe, Location was a term for the early African township, Harari Township, now called Mbare.
Mbuya	A term used to address an elderly woman, usually those above the age of fifty.
munyarikani	A respected person.
muroyi	Witch.
nyamukuta	Traditional midwife.
Rhodesian	This word is used to refer to white Zimbabweans during the colonial period.
sekuru	A term used to address an elderly male.
tete	Aunt.
urwere	Sickness.
zvirwerwe zvepabonde	Sexually transmitted diseases.

Bibliography

Archival material used

Africa University Archives

E. E. Bjorklund, Report of Medical Work at Old Umtali, Rhodesia Mission Conference, Methodist Episcopal Church, November 1926.
The Last Report of Dr Samuel Gurney to the Rhodesian Mission Conference, United Methodist Church, 19-25 June 1923.
Report of the Rhodesian Missionary Conference, United Methodist Church, 1909.
E. Sells, 'Medical practice between "two worlds"' (n.d.).

National Archives of Zimbabwe (NAZ)

Annual Report on the Public Health which covers Northern Rhodesia, Nyasaland and Southern Rhodesia, (1954).
F 242/SM/300/20 Nursing during the Federal Era.
F 242/SM/300/26 Southern Rhodesia Nurses' Association: From 1944. Government Notice No.335, 27 June 1927 (Government Printer: Salisbury, 1927).
LG 12/7/29 Resident Location Nurses. Entry into their quarters. 6 October 1944-18 March 1946.
LG 191/12/7/1 Native Welfare at the Location.
LG 191/12/7/88 Ante natal care: Illegal residents: Harari Township.
MS 308/38/1 Health Services in Relation to the Liberation Struggle.
MS 308/38/2 Health Services in Relation to the Liberation Struggle.
MS 308/38/3 Health Services in Relation to the Liberation Struggle. MS 308/38/4 Health Services in Relation to the Liberation Struggle.
Report of Public Health, 1939.
Report of Public Health, 1936.

Report of Public Health, 1941.
Report of Public Health, 1946.
Report of the Secretary for Health and Child Welfare for the year ending 31 December 1994.
Report of the Secretary for Health and Child Welfare for the year ending 31 December 1995.
Report of the Secretary for Health and Child Welfare for the year ending 31 December 1996.
Report of the Secretary for Health and Child Welfare for the year ending 31 December 1997.
Report of the Secretary for Health and Child Welfare for the year ending 31 December 1998.
Report of the Secretary for Health for the year ending 31 December 1966.
Report of the Secretary for Health for the year ending 31 December, 1974.
Report of the Secretary for Health for the year ended 31 December 1976.
Report of the Secretary for Health for the year ended 31 December 1977.
Report of the Secretary for Health for the year ending 31 December 1978.
S 1173/302 Chief Native Commissioner, Mission Stations.
S 119/1/2/1 Report of the Committee to Review Conditions of Services for Nurses in Government Employment, 1944.
S 2014/2/2 Shortage of Nursing Staff, 1940–1946.
S 2014/2/3 Recruitment, Nursing Staff, 1937–1939.
S 2014/23 Shortages of Nurses, 1940–1946.
S 2177/1/2 Nurses: General Correspondence, and Shortages of Nurses.
S 2177/3/1 Nurses: General Correspondence, and Shortages of Nurses.
S 2177/3/3 Salisbury Hospital: Correspondence: 1928–1948.
ZBI 2/1/2 The Howman Commission. The Report of the Committee to Investigate the Economic, Social and Health Condition of Africans Employed in Urban Areas (1944).
ZBP 1/2/4 National Health Services Commission.
ZBP 2/1/3 National Health Services Commission.

Periodicals and newspapers

The African Parade, June 1954.
The African Parade, June 1957.
The African Parade, August 1958.
The African Parade, November 1958.
The African Parade, January 1959.

Bibliography

The African Parade, February 1959.
The African Parade, September 1960.
The African Parade, December 1960.
The African Parade, April 1962.
The African Weekly, 4 January 1961.
The African Weekly, 25 January 1961
The African Weekly, 28 June 1961.
The African Weekly, 5 July 1961.
The African Weekly, 12 July 1961.
The Bantu Mirror, 11 July 1936.
The Bantu Mirror, 26 June 1937.
The Bantu Mirror, 24 December 1938.
The Bantu Mirror, 14 August 1942.
The Bantu Mirror, 16 October 1948.
The Herald, 25 October 1980.
The Herald, 22 October 1996.
The Herald, 23 October 1996.
The Herald, 24 October 1996.
The Herald, 30 October 1996.
The Herald, 31 October 1996.
The Herald, 1 November 1996.
The Herald, 12 November 1996.
The Herald, 15 November 1996.
The Herald, 21 November 1996.
The Herald, 7 October 2013.
Moto, June 1973.
Moto, June 1981.
The National Observer, 28 December 1978.
The Rhodesia Herald, 6 April 1973.
The Rhodesia Herald, 21 November 1974.
The Rhodesia Herald, 22 January 1975.
The Rhodesia Herald, 25 January 1975.
The Rhodesia Herald, 24 September 1977.
The Rhodesia Herald, 1 October 1977.
The Rhodesia Herald, 22 November 1978.
Rhodesia Parliamentary Debates, Vol. 91, 5–29 August 1975.
The Sunday Mail, 14 September 1980.
The Sunday Mail, 11 December 1983.
The Sunday Mail, 10 November 1996.

Bibliography

The Sunday Mail, 17 November 1996.
The Worker, February 1994.
The Worker, December–January 1995.
The Worker, March 1996.
The Zimbabwe Independent, 30 August–5 September 1996.
The Zimbabwe Independent, 15–21 November 1996. Parliamentary Debates.
Zimbabwe Parliamentary Debates, Vol. 2, 1980–1981, 19 August–8 October 1980, 20 January–7 May 1981.
Zimbabwe Parliamentary Debates, 27 November 1996.

Cited interviews by date

Brig. Gertrude Mutasa, *The Sunday Mail*, 11–16 February 2007. Interview by M. Mkwate.
Mrs Phaina Nyanhanda Harare, 15 August 2007. Interview by P. Mukwambo.
Mrs Fadzai Mugove, Harare, 10 July 2008.
Mrs Flora Matondo, Sakubva Mutare, 12 August 2008.
Mr Kufa Mutoro, Mutare, 12 August 2008.
Mrs D. Mtetwa, Mutare, 13 August 2008.
Mrs Estella Dhlamini, Harare, 22 August 2008.
Mrs Stella Munemo, Harare Hospital, 26 August 2008.
Mrs Noma Gudhlanga, Mutare, 28 August 2008.
Mrs Nhamo, Mufakose Harare, 13 September 2008.
Mrs Veronica Sibanda, Harare, 15 September 2008.
Mrs Dumbura, Mufakose Harare, 22 October 2008.
Mrs Laiza Shumba, Mabelreign Harare, 26 October 2008.
Mrs Mukono, Mabelreign Harare 27 October 2008.
Mrs Maida Tsopora, Harare, 28 October 2008.
Mrs Viola Moyo, Harare, 20 November 2008.
Mrs Doreen Mabika, Palmerstone Mutare, 4 January 2009.
Mrs Eneresia Makoto, Harare, 28 January 2009.
Mrs Esther Nyanhongo, Harare, 28 January 2009.
Mrs Maidei Madziwa, Sakubva Mutare, 10 February 2009.
Mrs Esther Mawoyo, Chikanga Mutare, 22 February 2009.
Mrs Wendy Mwamuka, Dangamvura Mutare, 17 April 2009.
Mrs Nomsa Makoni, Chitungwiza, 20 April 2009.
Mrs Nelia Ncube, Chitungwiza, 20 April 2009.
Mrs Jane Mushando, Sakubva Mutare, 27 April 2009.
Ms Tsitsi Chinamasa, Old Mutare, 28 May 2009.

Bibliography

Mrs Nyaradzo Buzengwe, Harare, 10 July 2009.
Mrs Christina Banda, Norton, July 2009.
Ms Claris Bere, Harare, July 2009. Interview by P. Mukwambo.
Brig. Felix Muchemwa, *The Sunday Mail*, 17-23 March 2013. Interview by M. Huni.
Mrs Viola Chirimuuta, Murehwa Mission, 3 May 2013. Interview by S. Machuma and recorded by G. Nera.
Akwino Aquous Muwoni, aka Texan Chidhakwa, *The Sunday Mail*, 5-11 May 2013. Interview by M. Huni.
Ms Marjorie M. Makaza, 17 April 2015, Mutare.
Rhodas Karimakwenda (nom de guerre - Anna Matambudziko), *The Sunday Mail*, 26 January - 1 February 2020. Interview by N. Muchemwa.

Articles, books and theses cited and for further reading

Agere, S. T., 'Progress and problems in the health care', in Mandaza, I (ed.), *Zimbabwe: The political economy of transition, 1980-1986* (Dakar: Codesria, 1986), pp. 355-76.

Alexander, J., J. McGregor and T. O. Ranger, *Violence and memory: One hundred years in the 'Dark Forests' of Matabeleland* (Harare: Weaver Press, 2000).

Apple, R., 'Afterword', in Sweet, H. and S. Hawkins (eds), *Colonial caring: A history of colonial and post-colonial nursing* (Manchester: Manchester University Press, 2015), pp. 232-6.

Arnold, D., 'Public health and public power: Medicine and hegemony in colonial India', in Engels, D. and S. Marks, *Contesting colonial hegemony: State and society in Africa and India* (New York: I.B. Taurus. 1994), pp. 131-50.

Aschwanden, H. (in collaboration with the African nursing sisters of Musiso Hospital, Zimbabwe), *Symbols of death: An analysis of the conscious of the Karanga* (Gweru: Mambo Press, 1987).

Barnes, T. A., '"So that a labourer could live with his family": Overlooked factors in the social and economic strife in urban colonial Zimbabwe, 1945-1952', *Journal of Southern African Studies*, 21: 1 (1995), pp. 95-113.

_____., *'We women worked so hard': Gender, urbanization and social reproduction in colonial Harare, Zimbabwe, 1930-1956* (Portsmouth, NH: Heinemann, 1999).

Barnes, T. A. and E. Win, *To live a better life: An oral history of women in the city of Harare, 1930-70* (Harare: Baobab Books, 1992).

Bell, H., 'Midwifery training and female circumcision in the interwar Anglo Egyptian Sudan', *Journal of African History*, 39: 2 (1998), pp. 292-312.

Bibliography

Benson, K. and J. M. Chadya, 'Ukubhinya: Gender and sexual violence in Bulawayo, colonial Zimbabwe, 1946-1956', *Journal of Southern African Studies*, 31: 3 (2005), pp. 587-610.

Berger, I., *Threads of solidarity: Women in South African industries* (Bloomington: Indiana University Press, 1992).

Bijlmakers, L. A., M. T. Bassett and D. M Sanders, 'Health and structural adjustment in rural and urban settings in Zimbabwe: Some interim findings', in Gibbon, P. (ed.), *Structural Adjustment and the working poor* (Uppsala: Nordiska Africainstitutet, 1995), pp. 215-82.

Birkett, D., 'The "white woman's burden" in the "white man's grave": Introduction of British nurses in colonial West Africa', in Chaudhuri, N. and M. Strobel (eds), *Western women and imperialism: Complicity and resistance* (Bloomington: Indiana University Press, 1992), pp. 177-88.

Bozzoli, B., 'Marxism, feminism and Southern African Studies', *Journal of Southern African Studies*, 9: 2 (1983), pp. 139-71.

Bryder, L., ' "They do what you wish; they like you the good nurse!": Colonialism and native health nursing in New Zealand, 1900-40', in Sweet, H. and S. Hawkins (eds), *Colonial caring: A history of colonial and post-colonial nursing* (Manchester: Manchester University Press, 2015), pp. 84-103.

Burke, T., *Lifebuoy men, Lux women: Commodification, consumption and cleanliness in modern Zimbabwe* (London: Routledge and Kegan Paul, 1996).

Burns, C., ' "A man is a clumsy thing who does not know how to handle a sick person": Aspects of the history of masculinity and race in the shaping of male nursing in South Africa, 1900-1950', *Journal of Southern African Studies*, 24: 4 (1998), pp. 695-717.

Catholic Commission for Justice and Peace, *Rhodesia: The propaganda war: Report prepared by the members of the Commission for Justice and Peace inside Rhodesia* (London: The Catholic Institute for International Relations, 1977).

Charumbira, R., 'Administering medicine without a license: Missionary women in Rhodesia's nursing history, 1890-1901', *The Historian*, 68: 2 (2006), pp. 241-66.

Cheru, F., *The silent revolution in Africa: Debt, development and democracy* (London: Zed Press, 1994).

Chidzero, B., 'The meaning of good government in Central Africa', in Leys, C. and C. Pratt (eds), *A new deal in Central Africa* (London: Heinemann, 1960), pp. 170-80.

Chikanda, A., 'Nurse migration from Zimbabwe: Analysis of recent trends and impacts', *Nursing Inquiry*, 12: 3 (2005), pp. 162-74.

Bibliography

Chipembere, E., 'Cross-border trade: A coping mechanism adopted by Zimbabweans: A case study of Harare, 1980-1999' (BA Honours Dissertation, University of Zimbabwe, 1999).

Choy, C. C., *Empire of care: Nursing and migration in Filipino American history* (Durham, NC and London: Duke University Press, 2003).

Clark Hine, D., *Black women in white: Racial conflict and cooperation in the nursing profession, 1890-1950* (Bloomington: Indiana University Press, 1989).

Clarke, D. G., *Agricultural and plantation workers in Rhodesia* (Salisbury: Mambo Press, 1977).

Cooper. F. and A. L. Stoler, *Tensions of empire: Colonial cultures in a bourgeoisie world* (Berkeley: University of California Press, 1997).

Craik, J., *Uniforms exposed: From conformity to transgression* (Oxford and New York: Berg, 2005).

Davies, C., *Rewriting nursing history* (Ottawa: Barnes and Nobles, 1980).

———, *Gender and the professional predicament of nursing* (Buckingham: Open University Press, 1996).

Digby, A. and H. Sweet, 'Nurses as cultural brokers in twentieth-century South Africa', in Ernst, W. (ed.), *Plural medicine, tradition and modernity, 1800-2000* (London and New York: Routledge, 2002), pp. 113-29.

Downie, G., 'Methodist Hospital, Nyadiri (Washburn Memorial) past and present', *Central African Journal of Medicine*, 8: 2 (1960), pp. 69-71.

Echenberg, M., *Africa in the time of cholera: A history of pandemic from 1815 to the present* (Cambridge: Cambridge University Press, 2011).

Etherington, N., 'Natal's black rape cases of the 1870s', *Journal of Southern African Studies*, 15: 1 (1988), pp. 36-53.

Fitzgerald, R., ' "Making and moulding the nursing of the Indian empire": Recasting nurses in colonial India', in Powell, A. A. and S. Lambert-Hurley (eds), *Rhetoric and reality: Gender and colonial experience in South Asia* (Oxford: Oxford University Press, 2006) pp. 185-222.

Fraser Ross, W., 'The Advanced Clinical Nurse', *Central African Journal of Medicine*, 22: 3 (1976) pp. 56-7.

———, 'Nursing in Rhodesia, past, present and future', *Rhodesia Nurse*, (1967), p. 32.

Frederiske, J., *None but ourselves: Masses and media in the making of Zimbabwe* (New York: Penguin Books, 1984).

Gaidzanwa, R., *Voting with their feet: Migrant Zimbabwean nurses and doctors in the era of structural adjustment* (Uppsala: Nordiska Afrikainstitutet, 1999).

Gamble, V., *Making a place for ourselves: The black hospital movement, 1920-1945* (Oxford: Oxford University Press, 1995).

Bibliography

Garmarnikow, E., 'Sexual division of labor: The case of nursing', in Kuhn, A. and A. M. Wolpe (eds), *Feminism and materialism: Women and modes of production* (London: Boston and Henley, 1978), pp. 96–123.

Gear, H. S., 'Some problems of the medical services of the Federation of Rhodesia and Nyasaland', *British Medical Journal*, 2 (1960), pp. 525–31.

Gelfand, M., *Tropical victory: An account of the influence of medicine on the history of Southern Rhodesia, 1890–1923* (Cape Town: Juta, 1953).

———, *A proud record: An account of the health services provided for Africans in the Federation of Rhodesia and Nyasaland* (Salisbury: Government Printer, 1960).

———, *A service to the sick: A history of the health services for Africans in Southern Rhodesia.1890–1953* (Gwelo: Mambo Press, 1976).

———, 'Harare Hospital ('Gomo') comes of age', *Central African Journal of Medicine*, 25: 8 (1979), pp. 177–8.

Giles-Vernick, T., 'Oral histories as methods and sources', in Perecman, E. and S. R. Currran, *Handbook for Social Science field research: Essays and bibliographic sources on research design and methods* (Thousand Oaks, CA: Sage Publications, 2006), pp. 85–95.

Gillmurray, J., R. Riddel and D. Sanders, *The struggles for health from Rhodesia to Zimbabwe* (London: Catholic Institute for International Relations, 1979).

Govha, C., 'A study of the implications of racial and gender prejudices on African women in the nursing profession in colonial Zimbabwe, 1890–1960' (BA Honours, University of Zimbabwe, 2001).

Gray, R., *The two nations: Aspects of the development of race relations in Rhodesia and Nyasaland* (London: Oxford University Press, 1960).

Hardiman, D., 'Introduction', in Hardiman, D. (ed.), *Healing bodies, saving souls: Medical missions in Asia and Africa* (Amsterdam: Rodopi, 2006), pp. 5–57.

Horwitz, S., '"Black nurses in white": Exploring young women's entry into the nursing profession at Baragwanath Hospital, Soweto, 1948–1980', *Social History Medicine*, 20: 1 (2007), pp. 131–46.

———, *Baragwanath Hospital Soweto: A History of Medical Care 1941–1990* (Johannesburg: Wits University Press, 2013).

Hunt, N. R., *A colonial lexicon: Of birth ritual, medicalization, and mobility in the Congo* (Durham. NC: Duke University Press, 1999).

Illife, J., *East African doctors: A history of the modern profession* (Cambridge: Cambridge University Press, 1998).

Isaacman A. F. and B. Isaacman, *Dams, displacement, and the delusion of development* (Pietermaritzburg: University of Natal Press, 2013).

Bibliography

Jackson, L., "When in the white man's town": Zimbabwean women remember chibeura', in Allman, J., S. Geiger and N. Musisi (eds), *Women in African colonial histories* (Bloomington: Indiana University Press, 2002) pp. 191–215.

―――, *Surfacing up: Psychiatry and social order in colonial Zimbabwe* (Ithaca, NY: Cornell University Press, 2005).

Janzen, J., *The quest for therapy: Medical pluralism in lower Zaire* (Berkeley: University of California Press, 1978).

Jeater, D., *Marriage, perversion, and power: The construction of moral discourse in Southern Rhodesia, 1894–1930* (Oxford: Clarendon Press, 1993).

Johnson, D., *World War Two and the scramble for labor in colonial Zimbabwe, 1939–1948* (Harare: University of Zimbabwe Publications, 2000).

Kaler, A., *Running after their pills: Politics, gender and contraception in colonial Zimbabwe* (Portsmouth, NH: Heinemann, 2003).

Kalusa, W. T., 'Language, medical auxiliaries, and the reinterpretation of missionary medicine in colonial Mwinilunga, Zambia, 1922–1951', *The Journal of Eastern African Studies*, 1: 1 (2007), pp. 57–78.

Kavumbura, B. J. and R. T. Mossop, 'Attitudes to Illness in Salisbury, 1980', *Central African Journal of Medicine*, 26: 5 (1980), pp. 111–14.

Khan, N. and N. Jazdowska, 'Women, workers and discrimination in Zimbabwe', in Raftopoulos, B. and L. Sachikonye (eds), *Striking Back: The labour movement and the post-colonial state in Zimbabwe, 1980–2000* (Harare: Weaver Press, 2001), pp. 175–96.

Landau, P., *The realm of the word: Language, gender and Christianity in a southern African kingdom* (Portsmouth, NH: James Currey. 1995).

Lela, J. W. and D. Pawluch, 'Medical students and the cadaver in social and cultural context', in Lock, M. and D. Gordon (eds), *Biomedicine examined* (London: Kluver Academic Publishers, 1988), pp. 125–53.

Levy, L. F., 'Keeping abreast of the times', *Central African Journal of Medicine*, 8: 2 (1962), pp. 158–9.

Leys, C., ' "Partnership" as the dismantling of colour bar', in Leys, C. and C. Pratt (eds), *A new deal in Central Africa* (London: Heinemann, 1960), pp. 98–109.

Leys, C. and C. Pratt (eds), *A new deal in Central Africa* (London: Heinemann, 1960).

Loewenson, R., D. Sanders and R. Davies, 'Challenges to equity in health and health care: A Zimbabwean case study', *Social Science & Medicine*, 32: 10 (1991), pp. 1079–88.

Lubanga, N., 'Nursing in South Africa: Black women workers organize', in Turshen, M. (ed.), *Women and health in Africa* (Trenton: Africa World Press, 1991), pp. 51–77.

Bibliography

McClintock, A., *Imperial leather: Race, gender and sexuality in colonial conquest* (New York: Routledge, 1995).

McCulloch, J., *Black peril, white virtue: Sexual crime in Southern Rhodesia, 1902–1935* (Bloomington: Indiana University Press, 2000).

_____, *Asbestos blues: Labour, capital, physicians and the state in South Africa* (Oxford: James Currey, 2002).

MacGaffey, J., 'Evading male control: Women in the second economy of Zaire', in Stichter, S. and J. Parpart (eds), *Patriarchy and class: African women in the home and the workplace* (Boulder, CO: Westview Press, 1988), pp. 161–76.

McGregor, J., 'Professionals relocating: Zimbabwean nurses and teachers negotiating work and family in Britain', Geographical Paper, 178, *Geography* (2006), (University of Reading, UK).

McLaughlin, J., *On the frontline: Catholic missions in Zimbabwe liberation war* (Baobab Books: Harare, 1996).

Made, P. A., and N. Whande, 'Women in Southern Africa: A note on the Zimbabwean "success story"', *Issue: A Journal of Opinion*, 17: 2 (1989), pp. 26–8.

Marks, S., *Divided sisterhood: Race, class and gender in the South African nursing profession* (London: St Martin's Press, 1994).

_____, 'What is colonial about colonial medicine? And what has happened to imperialism and health?', *Social History of Medicine*, 10: 2 (2002), pp. 205–19.

_____, '"We were men nursing men": Male nursing on the mines in twentieth-century South Africa', in Woodward, W., P. Hayes and G. Minkley (eds), *Deep histories: Gender and colonialism in Southern Africa* (Amsterdam: Rodipi, 2002), pp. 177–204.

Marks, S. and N. Anderson, 'Industrialization, rural health and the National Health Service Commission in South Africa', in Feierman, S. and J. Janzen (eds), *The social basis of health and healing in Africa* (Berkeley: University of California Press, 1992), pp. 131–74.

Martinez, I., 'The history of the use of bacteriological and chemical agents during Zimbabwe's liberation war of 1965–80 by Rhodesian Forces', *Third World Quarterly*, 23: 6 (2002), pp. 1159–79.

Masakure, C., '"One of the most serious problems confronting us at present": Nurses and government hospitals in Southern Rhodesia, 1930s to 1950', *Historia*, 60: 2 (2015), pp. 109–31.

_____, 'The politicisation of health in Zimbabwe: The case of the cholera epidemic, August 2008 – March 2009', *New Contree*, 80 (2018), pp. 65–88.

_____, 'Government hospitals as a microcosm: Integration and segregation in Salisbury Hospital, Rhodesia, 1890s–1950', in Stevens Crawshaw,

Bibliography

J. L., I. Benyovsky Latin and K. Vongsathorn (eds), *Tracing hospital boundaries: Integration and segregation in Southeastern Europe and beyond, 1050–1970* (Brill: Leiden, 2020), pp. 246–69.

Mashaba, G., *The rising challenge: A history of black nursing in South Africa* (Cape Town: Juta, 1995).

Mavhunga, C. C., 'Guerrilla healthcare innovation: Creative resilience in Zimbabwe's Chimurenga, 1971–1980', *History and Technology*, 31: 3 (2015), p. 301.

Maxwell, D., *Christian and chiefs in Zimbabwe: A social history of the Hwesa c.1870s–1990s* (London: Edinburgh University Press. 1999).

Melchior, F., 'Feminist approaches to nursing history', *Western Journal of Nursing Research*, 26: 3 (2004), pp. 340–55.

Melosh, B., *The physician's hand: Work, culture and conflict in American nursing* (Philadelphia, PA: Temple University Press, 1982).

Mhike, I., 'A perennial shortage: State Registered Nurse training and recruitment in Southern Rhodesia's government hospitals, 1939–1963' (MA dissertation, University of Zimbabwe, 2007).

Mlambo, A., *The Economic Structural Adjustment Programme: The case of Zimbabwe, 1990–1995* (Harare: University of Zimbabwe Publication, 1997).

Mnyanda, B. J., *In search of truth: A commentary on certain aspects of Southern Rhodesian Native Policy* (Hind Kitabs: Bombay, 1954).

Moorcroft, P. L. and McLaughlin, P., *The Rhodesian war: Fifty years on* (Barnsley: Pen and Sword Books Ltd, 2015).

Msipa, C. G., *In pursuit of freedom and justice: A memoir* (Harare: Weaver Press, 2015).

Munyaradzi, O. M. and C. Muronda, 'Some attitudes of patients discharged from Harare Hospital', *Central African Journal of Medicine*, 25: 5 (1979), pp. 104–7.

Mutizwa-Mangiza, D., *Doctors and the state: The struggle for professional control in Zimbabwe* (Aldershot: Ashgate, 1999).

Ncube, G., 'The making of rural healthcare in colonial Zimbabwe: A history of the Ndanga Medical Unit, Fort Victoria, 1930–1960s' (PhD thesis, Department of Historical Studies, University of Cape Town, 2012).

Nzenza, S., *Zimbabwean woman: My own story* (London: Karia Press, 1988).

O'Gorman, E., *The front line runs through every woman: Women and local resistance in the Zimbabwean War* (London: James Carrey, 2011).

Packard, R., *White plague, black labor: Tuberculosis and the political economy of health and disease in South Africa* (Berkeley: University of California Press, 1989).

Pape, J., 'Black and white: The "perils of sex" in colonial Zimbabwe', *Journal of Southern African Studies*, 16: 4 (1990), pp. 699–720.

―――, 'Still serving the tea: Domestic workers in Zimbabwe 1980', *Journal of Southern African Studies*, 19: 3 (1993), pp. 387–404.

―――, 'Changing education for majority rule in Zimbabwe and South Africa', *Comparative Education Review*, 42: 3 (1998), pp. 253–66.

Parle, J. and V. Noble, *The people's hospital: A history of McCord, Durban, 1890s–1970s* (Pietermaritzburg: Natal Society Foundation, 2018).

Payer, C., *The debt trap: The International Monetary Fund and the Third World* (New York: Monthly Review Press, 1974).

Phimister, I. R., 'The "Spanish" influenza pandemic of 1918 and its impact on the Southern Rhodesian mining industry', *Central African Journal of Medicine*, 19: 7 (1973), pp. 143–8.

―――, 'African labour conditions and health in Southern Rhodesian mining industry, 1898–1953. Part IV: Hospitalisation and conclusions', *Central African Journal of Medicine*, 22: 12 (1976), pp. 244–9.

―――, *An economic and social history of Zimbabwe: Capital accumulation and class struggle* (London: Cambridge University Press, 1988).

Physicians for Human Rights, *Health in ruins: A man-made disaster in Zimbabwe* (Cambridge, MA: Physicians for Human Rights, 2008/9).

Raftopoulos, B., 'The crisis in Zimbabwe, 1998–2008', in Raftopoulos, B., and A. Mlambo (eds), *Becoming Zimbabwe: A history from the pre-colonial period to 2008* (Harare: Weaver Press, 2009), pp. 201–32.

Raftopoulos, B. and I. R. Phimister (eds), *Keep on knocking: A history of labour movement in Zimbabwe* (Harare: Baobab Books, 1997).

Raftopoulos, B. and L. Sachikonye, *Striking back: The labour movement and the post-colonial state in Zimbabwe, 1980–2000* (Harare: Weaver Press, 2001).

Ranger, T. O., 'The influenza pandemic in Southern Rhodesia: A crisis of comprehension', in Arnold, D. (ed.), *Imperial Medicine and indigenous societies* (Manchester: Manchester University Press, 1988), pp. 172–88.

―――, 'Dignifying death: The politics of burial in Bulawayo', *The Journal of Religion in Africa*, 34: 1–2 (2004), pp. 110–44.

―――, *Bulawayo burning: A social history of a Southern African town, 1893–1960* (Harare: Weaver Press, 2010).

Ransford, O., *Bid the sickness cease: Disease in the history of black Africa* (London: John Murray, 1983).

Ray, S. and F. Madzimbamuto, 'The HIV epidemic in Zimbabwe: The penalty of silence', *The Round Table*, 95: 384 (2006), pp. 219–38.

Reverby, S., *Ordered to care: The dilemma of American nursing, 1850–1945* (New York: Cambridge University Press, 1987).

Bibliography

Rittey, D. A. W., 'The story of a leprosy patient', *Central African Journal of Medicine*, 18: 11 (1972), pp. 230–2.

Roberts, R., *Litigants and households: African disputes and colonial courts in the French Soudan, 1895-1912* (Portsmouth, NH: Heinemann, 2005).

Ross, L. J., 'African-American women and abortion: A neglected history', *Journal of Health Care for the Poor and Underserved*, 3: 2 (1992), pp. 274–84.

Rubert, S., *A most promising weed: A history of tobacco farming and labor in colonial Zimbabwe, 1890-1945* (Cleveland: Ohio University Press, 1998).

Sandelowski, M., *Devices and desires: Gender, technology, and American nursing* (Chapel Hill and London. The University of North Carolina Press, 2000).

Sanders, D., 'Equity in health: Zimbabwe nine years on', *Journal of Social Development in Africa*, 5: 1 (1990) 5–22.

Sanders, R., 'Striking ahead: Industrial action and labour movement development in Zimbabwe', in Raftopoulos, B. and L. Sachikonye (eds), *Striking back: The labour movement and the post-colonial state in Zimbabwe, 1980-2000* (Harare: Weaver Press, 2001), pp. 133–74.

Schmidt, E., *Peasants, traders and wives: Shona women in the history of Zimbabwe, 1870-1939* (Heinemann, NH: Portsmouth, 1992).

Sedman, G. W., 'Women in Zimbabwe: Post independence struggles', *Feminist Studies*, 10: 3 (1984), pp. 419–40.

Sells, E., 'Medical Practice between "Two Worlds": A woman tells how Dr Gurney put back her intestines', *Rhodesia – the Methodist Church – Yesterday and Today* (Africa University Archives, no date but likely published in the 1960s).

Shutt, A., 'Litigating honor, defamation, and shame in Southern Rhodesia', *African Studies Review*, 61: 3 (2018), pp. 79–98.

Shutt, A. K., *Manners make a nation: Racial etiquette in Southern Rhodesia, 1910-1963* (Rochester, NY: University of Rochester Press, 2015).

Simmons, D., 'Religion and medicine at the crossroads: A re-examination of the Southern Rhodesian influenza epidemic of 1918', *Journal of Southern African Studies*, 35: 1 (2009), pp. 29–44.

Smith, S. L., *Sick and tired of being sick and tired: Black women's health activism in America, 1890-1950* (Philadelphia: University of Pennsylvania Press, 1995).

Stapleton, T., *African police and soldiers in colonial Zimbabwe, 1923-1980* (Rochester: University of Rochester Press, 2011).

Staunton, I. (ed.), *Mothers of the revolution: The war experiences of thirty women in Zimbabwe* (London: James Carrey, 1990).

Stichter, S. B., 'The middle-class family in Kenya: Changes in gender relations', in Stichter, S. B. and J. Parpart (eds), *Patriarchy and class: African women in the home and workplace* (Boulder, CO: Westview Press, 1995), pp. 177–203.

Bibliography

Stoler, A. and F. Cooper, 'Between metropole and colony: Rethinking a research agenda', in Stoler, A. and F. Cooper (eds), *Tensions of empire: Colonial cultures in a bourgeois world* (Berkeley: University of California Press, 1997), pp. 1–56.

Summers, C., *Colonial lessons: Africans' education in Southern Rhodesia, 1918–1940* (Oxford: James Currey, 2002).

Swaisland, C., *Servants and gentlewomen to the golden land: The emigration of single women from Britain to southern Africa, 1820–1939* (Pietermaritzburg: University of Natal Press, 1993).

Sweet, H., 'Mission nursing in South African context: The spread of knowledge during the colonial and apartheid eras', in Fleischmann, E., S. Grypma, M. Marten and I. M. Okkenhaug (eds), *Transnational and historical perspectives on global health, welfare and humanitarianism* (Kristiansand: Portal Forlag Publishers, 2013), pp. 137–57.

Sweet, H. and A. Digby, 'Race, identity and nursing profession in South Africa, c.1850–1958', in Mortimer, B. and S. McGann (eds), *New direction in nursing history: International perspectives* (Routledge: New York, 2005), pp. 109–24.

Sweet, H. and S. Hawkins (eds), *Colonial caring: A history of colonial and postcolonial nursing* (Manchester: Manchester University Press, 2015).

Thomas, L., *The politics of the womb: Women, reproduction and the state in Kenya* (Berkeley: University of California Press, 2003).

Tripp, A. M., 'Deindustrialization and the growth of women's economic associations and networks in urban Tanzania', in Rowbotham, S. and S. Mitter (eds), *Dignity and daily bread: New forms of economic organizing among poor women into the Third World and the First* (London: Penguin, 1994), pp. 139–57.

Trouillot, M., *Silencing the past: Power and the production of history* (Boston, MA: Beacon Press. 1995).

Turrittin, J., 'Colonial midwives and modernizing childbirth in French West Africa', in Allman, J., S. Geiger and N. Musisi (eds), *Women in African colonial histories* (Bloomington: Indiana University Press, 2002), pp. 71–90.

Turshen, M., *The political ecology of disease in Tanzania* (New Brunswick, NJ: Rutgers University Press, 1984).

Ushewokunze, H. S. M., *An agenda for Zimbabwe* (Harare: College Press, 1984).

Van Onselen, C., *Chibaro: African mine labour in Southern Rhodesia, 1900–1933* (London: Pluto Press, 1976).

Vaughan, M., *Curing their ills: Colonial power and African illness* (Stanford, CA: Stanford University Press, 1991).

Vera, Y., *Butterfly burning* (Harare: Baobab Books, 1998).

Wall, B. M., *Into Africa: A transnational history of Catholic medical missions and social change* (New Brunswick, NJ: Rutgers University Press, 2015).

Bibliography

Warhurst, P. R., 'The history of race relations in Rhodesia', *Zambezia*, 3: 1 (1973), pp. 15–19.

Weinrich, A. K. H., *Black and white rural elites in Rhodesia* (Manchester: Manchester University Press, 1973).

West, M., *The rise of an African middle class: Colonial Zimbabwe, 1898-1965* (Bloomington: Indiana University Press, 2002).

White, L., *Speaking with vampires: Rumor and history in colonial Africa* (Berkeley: University of California Press, 2000).

Whitehead, J., 'The Andrew Fleming Hospital, Salisbury, Rhodesia', *Annals of the Royal College of Surgeons of England*, 54 (1974), pp. 313–14.

Wilkinson, A. R., 'The impact of the war', in Morris-Jones, W. H. (ed.), *From Rhodesia to Zimbabwe: Behind and beyond Lancaster House* (London: Frank Cass, 1980), pp. 110–23.

Yoshikuni, T., *African urban experiences in colonial Zimbabwe: A social history of Harare before 1925* (Harare: Weaver Press, 2007).

ZANU-PF, *Zimbabwe at 5 years of independence: Achievements, problems and prospects* [Preface: R. G. Mugabe] (Harare: ZANU (PF) Department of Commissariat and Culture, 1985).

Zelnick, J., and M. O'Donnell, 'The impact of HIV/AIDS epidemic on hospital nurses in KwaZulu Natal, South Africa', *Journal of Public Health Policy*, 26: 2 (2005), pp. 163–85.

Zimudzi, T. B., 'African women, violent crime and the criminal law in colonial Zimbabwe, 1900–1952', *Journal of Southern African Studies*, 30: 3 (2004), pp. 499–517.

Index

abortion 109
Advanced Clinical Nurse 150, 217
Advanced Male Native Nursing Orderlies 5, 25, 41, 47, 53, 217
African middle class 7, 13, 14, 48, 65, 77, 81, 87, 88, 152, 194
African patients
  close contact with white women 50, 51
  explanation of illness 5, 6, 114, 118, 119
  translation of biomedicine to 4, 9, 119, 120
Africanisation of hospitals 3, 94, 95, 96, 127, 136, 183, 206, 217, 220
Africanisation of nursing services 94, 95, 101, 127, 128, 137, 214
Asian
  nurses of Asian descent 3, 16, 53, 54, 73, 83, 94, 98, 99, 127, 137, 138, 139, 141, 216, 222
Askins, Robert A. 41

Banda, Christina 70, 125, 126
Barnes, Teresa 80
Ben, Barbara 36
Bere, Claris 193
Bilharzia 44, 116, 148, 151
birth control 109
Bjorklund, E. 33

'Black Peril' scares 51
Burns, Catherine 50, 221
Bush hospitals 11, 137, 167
Buzengwe, Nyaradzo 115, 118

cadaver experiences 124, 126, 127
certified nurses 34, 35
Chieza, Constance 39
Chinamasa, Tsitsi 71, 76
cholera epidemic 14, 17
choosing nursing as a career option 7, 9, 64, 65, 67, 75, 88, 219
colonial medicine 4, 6, 96, 119, 215, 218
coloured nurses 3, 16, 50, 53, 54, 63, 73, 83, 94, 98, 99, 104, 127, 137, 138, 139, 142, 216, 222
coping strategies (1990s) 11, 174, 192, 194, 220
coping strategies to assert independence 108
cross-border trading 195, 206
cultural brokers, nurses as 4, 118, 119, 121, 122, 218
cultural interlocutors, nurses as 4, 5, 218

Democratic Republic of Congo 121
Denga, Naomi 39
Dhlamini, Estella 15, 17, 195, 197

Index

diarrhoea 30, 150, 160
Digby, Anne 4, 50
dispensary 26, 31, 35, 42
Dry, Madge Sr 36, 37, 215
dysentery 29, 30, 160

Economic Structural Adjustment Programme 188, 193, 195, 206, 220

Federal Nursing Service 102, 103
Fleming, Andrew 34, 36, 41

Gelfand, Michael 36, 42, 44, 49, 63
generational differences amongst nurses 16, 76, 107
Gezi, Annie 39
Gothosa, Julius 42
Gudhlanga, Noma 152, 155, 156
Gunapira, David 42
Gurney, Samuel 5, 26, 28, 29, 124

Harari Township
  location 48, 77, 78, 79, 111
  location clinic 48, 49, 50, 77, 111
Hawkins, Sue 4, 8
history of hospitals 1, 15
HIV/AIDS 11, 17, 174, 188, 190, 191, 192, 206, 220
Horwitz, S. 9, 64
hospitals
  Andrew Fleming Hospital 140
  Barrage Military Hospital, Mozambique 165
  Bindura Hospital 138
  Bonda Mission Hospital 40, 117
  Bulawayo General Hospital 49, 99
  Chibi Rural Hospital 148
  Chimoio Hospital 157
  closure of 17, 198, 200, 203
  culture of 7, 118
  desegregation of 11, 175, 176
  Gwelo General Hospital 178, 179
  Harare Hospital 14, 52, 186
  Harari Hospital 6, 63, 88, 94, 99, 102, 103, 108, 147
  hierarchical nature of 3, 73, 95, 105
  Hospital Police Boys 30
  Howard Mission Hospital 38
  impact of HIV/AIDS pandemic on 192
  Impilo Hospital 63, 87, 88, 94, 99, 102, 103
  Ingutsheni Hospital 47
  McCord Hospital, South Africa 63, 94, 100
  mining centres 30
  Mnene Mission Hospital 38
  Morgenster Mission Hospital 37, 148
  Mpilo Hospital 52
  Mt Selinda Mission Hospital 37
  Mtoko Medical Unit 41
  Ndanga Medical Unit 41
  Nyadiri Mission Hospitals 38
  Old Umtali Mission Hospital 26, 33
  Parirenyatwa Bush Hospital 157, 161
  Parirenyatwa Hospital 14
  Princess Margaret Hospital 63, 88, 94, 98
  Salisbury General Hospital 12, 43, 48, 49
  sites of struggles 9, 10
  struggles within 2
  Umtali General Hospital 47, 94
  Waddilove Mission Hospital 36, 37, 40
Hunt, Nancy Rose 4, 118

Illife, John 127
influenza pandemic 30, 31, 32, 53

Kennedy, James 41
Kenya 42
Kudzai, Rebecca 38

Index

Labour Relations Act 185
Legate, James 41
leprosy 27, 148, 214
Levy, Laurence Fraser 139, 140, 142

Mabika, Doreen 182, 191
Madenyika, Grace 38
Madeya, Titus 42
Madziwa, Maidei 75
Magole, James 42
Majeke, Miriam 39
Makaza, Marjorie 157, 158, 159, 160
Maketo, Esther 36
Makoni, Makoni 72
Makoni, Nomsa 18, 71, 177, 183, 187
Makoto, Eneresia 145, 146, 147
malaria 29, 33, 44, 116, 148, 151, 165
male nurses 10, 12, 35, 36, 44, 221, 222
malnutrition 17, 150, 160, 207
Manawana, Monica 39
Manyoka, Jonathan 27, 216
Marange, Margaret 39
Marks, Shula 8, 50, 51, 52, 73, 174, 197
Martin, Andrew Paton 42
Maseko, Martin 43
maternity leave 183, 184, 185
Matondo, Flora 5, 102, 113, 119, 140, 190
Mawoyo, Estha 72, 73, 76, 112
medical assistants 24, 27, 32, 33, 41, 44, 149
medical auxiliaries 24, 27, 29, 32, 46, 47, 53, 214, 216
Medical Council of Rhodesia 41, 42
medical grant 25, 34, 36
medics 10, 11, 137, 158, 160, 161, 162, 163, 164, 165, 166, 217, 221, 223
Melosh, Barbara 7, 8, 106
Mgugu, Dinah 36
Mhlope, Robinson Tholana 42

midwifery 36, 37, 38, 63, 67, 96, 97, 100, 113, 138, 165
midwives 42, 47, 50, 94, 96, 97, 127, 216
Moyo, Marty 38
Moyo, Miriam Dhlembeu 39, 117, 123
Mtetwa, D. 151
Muchemwa, Felix 160, 161, 162
Mugabe, Robert 175, 179, 199
Mugove, Fadzai 114
Muhango, Godfrey 44
Musa, Richard 43
Mushando, Jane 74, 75, 112, 122, 123, 192, 193
Mutasa, Getrude 158, 159, 162, 165
Mutoro, Kufa 24, 46, 67
Muwoni, Akwino Aquous 160, 161, 163, 164, 165
Mwamuka, Wendy 66, 67
Myambe, E. 43

National Health Services Commission 12, 13, 50, 116, 124
Ncube, Nelia 72, 83, 143, 183, 184
Neves, Tizora M. 27
Nguni, Simon 43
night duty 76, 83, 110, 112, 132, 144, 183, 184, 195
Nirdjesjo, Plof W. 52
Nondo, Clara 189, 197
Northern Rhodesia 63, 70
nurse aides 47, 94, 127
nurse-patient relationships 6, 118, 121, 186, 191, 214
nurses' autonomy 3, 4, 44, 105, 151
nurses' uniforms 72, 73, 120, 125
nursing assistants 3, 24, 25, 35, 53, 68, 70, 71, 77, 78, 79, 116, 117, 124, 158
nursing history
general 4, 8, 219, 220, 222, 223
South Africa 9

Index

Zimbabwe 9, 10, 18, 221
nursing orderlies 3, 10, 24, 25, 27, 40, 41, 42, 43, 44, 46, 47, 50, 52, 53, 54, 67, 70, 71, 78, 82, 115, 116, 124, 125, 146, 159, 163, 197, 198, 214, 215, 216, 217, 221, 223
nursing prestige 1, 2, 64, 70, 71, 82, 122
nursing professional identity 64, 70, 71, 72, 74, 76, 77, 89, 112, 118, 127
Nyanhanda, Phaina 15, 80, 84, 85, 125
Nyanhongo, Esther 149, 150
Nyasaland 42, 63, 101, 104

Page, Sr Lorna 39, 40
pneumonia 29, 151
pregnancy 85, 108, 150, 176, 184
probationer nurse 35, 36, 38

qualified nurse 25, 36, 48, 52, 83, 95, 101, 108, 112, 139, 216

Rhoades, Helen Barbara 63
rural nurses during the war 10, 136, 157, 166

Sabangana, Eva 38
Sadomba, R. T. D. 142
Sakutomba, David 33, 34, 46, 216
salaries 16, 35, 36, 58, 82, 83, 84, 85, 88, 101, 143, 185, 192, 194, 201, 204, 205, 206, 220
scabies 150
sexually transmitted diseases 17, 18, 29, 53, 160
Shumba, Laiza 1, 2, 18, 74, 75, 86, 96, 102, 107, 112, 122, 154, 189
Sibanda, Howard 43
Sibanda, Veronica 120, 198
Sidambe, Timothy 43
silicosis 30

Sloman, Sr 38
smallpox 29, 44
social mobility of nurses 6, 7, 65
Southern Rhodesia Nurses' Association 12
Southern Rhodesian Missionary Conference 34, 36
SRN *see* State Registered Nurse 188
Stamps, Timothy 188
State Registered Nurse (SRN) 7, 25, 40, 48, 49, 50, 52, 54, 63, 64, 88, 97, 98, 99, 100, 103, 104, 108, 139, 216, 217, 222
Stokvels 194
strikes 18, 196, 197, 198, 199, 200, 201, 203, 204, 205, 207, 220, 222
Sweet, Helen 4, 8, 50

training
  of Advanced Clinical Nurses 36
  age to commence training at mission hospitals 36
  of coloured nurses 54
  of coloured nurses at Bulawayo General Hospital 99
  of coloured nurses at Princess Margaret Hospital 63, 88, 94
  of male nurses 10, 12, 48, 52
  of medical auxiliaries 34, 35
  of medics during the war 159, 160, 162
  of microscopists 47
  of midwives at mission hospitals 36
  of midwives at Umtali General Hospital 94
  number of nurses training at mission hospitals in 1943 39
  of nurse aides 47, 94
  of nurses 10, 49, 53
  of nurses at Bonda Mission Hospital 39
  of nurses at Harari Hospital 63, 88, 94

Index

of nurses at Howard Mission Hospital 38
of nurses at Impilo Hospital 63, 88, 94
of nurses at mission hospitals 5, 25, 33, 41
of nurses at Mnene Mission Hospital 38
of nurses at Morgenster Mission Hospital 37, 38
of nurses at Mt Selinda Mission Hospital 37
of nurses at Nyadiri Mission Hospital 38
of nurses at Waddilove Mission Hospital 37
of nurses of Asian descent 54
of nurses of Asian descent at Bulawayo General Hospital 99
of nurses of Asian descent at Princess Margaret Hospital 94
of nursing orderlies 25, 41, 42, 43
Preliminary Training School 110
public complaints on student nurses at Harari Hospital 108
of Rhodesian nurses at McCord Hospital, South Africa 94, 100
of Rhodesian nurses in South Africa 88
of State Registered Nurses 49, 50, 52, 97
years of training at mission hospitals 35

Tsiga, Job 5, 28, 29, 34, 46, 216
tuberculosis 17, 30, 113
Tyeza, Lilian 36
typhoid 29

urban nurses during the war 10, 136, 147, 148, 166
Ushewokunze, Herbert 157, 173, 176, 177, 178, 179, 181, 183

Vaughan, Megan 9, 26, 27
venereal diseases 29, 44
Victorian ideology 52, 66, 81

war casualties, nursing of 136, 148
white (European) nurses 3, 7, 9, 12, 36, 37, 49, 50, 51, 83, 97, 99, 101, 102, 104, 105, 136, 137, 138, 139, 140, 142, 143, 145, 146, 149, 152, 166, 182, 206, 217, 219, 222
white medical personnel 4, 46, 128, 218
witchcraft 5, 113, 124, 126, 204
workplace relations 2, 3, 7, 8, 9, 73, 95, 105, 106, 128, 144, 180, 183, 203, 217

Zimbabwe Congress of Trade Unions 202
Zimbabwe Nurses Association 189, 197

EU authorised representative for GPSR:
Easy Access System Europe, Mustamäe tee 50,
10621 Tallinn, Estonia
gpsr.requests@easproject.com